Contents

List of tables and figures

Tables

Figures

Acknowledgements

The authors are grateful to the Economic and
Social Research Council (ESRC) Data Archive at
Essex for access to data from the 1958 to 1991
National Child Development Study (NCDS).

We would also like to thank David Riley, the
nominated officer at the Department of the
Environment, Transport and the Regions, for his
advice and comments during the project, Alan
Holmans of Cambridge University for his
comments on earlier drafts of this report, and Peter
Shepherd of the Centre for Longitudinal Studies,
Institute of Education for his assistance. Ray Forrest
provided valuable assistance during the project and
comments on the report. The three anonymous
referees for The Policy Press and Lyn Harrison also
provided valuable comments and suggestions.

Any remaining errors of fact or interpretation are
the responsibility of the authors alone.

Home Sweet Home?

The impact of poor housing on health

Alex Marsh, David Gordon, Christina Pantazis
and Pauline Heslop

First published in Great Britain in 1999 by

The Policy Press
University of Bristol
Fourth Floor, Beacon House
Queen's Road
Bristol BS8 1QU
UK

Tel   +44 (0)117 331 4054
Fax   +44 (0)117 331 4093
E-mail tpp-info@bristol.ac.uk
www.policypress.org.uk

Transferred to Digital Print 2008

ISBN 978 1 86134 1 76 1

Alex Marsh is Lecturer in Urban Studies, School for Policy Studies, **David Gordon** is a Research Fellow at the School for Policy Studies, **Christina Pantazis** is a Research Fellow at the School for Policy Studies and **Pauline Heslop** is a researcher at the Department of Social Medicine, all at the University of Bristol.

The right of Alex Marsh, David Gordon, Christina Pantazis and Pauline Heslop to be identified as authors of this work have been asserted by them in accordance with Sections 77 and 78 of the 1988 Copyright, Designs and Patents Act.

The statements and opinions contained within this publication are solely those of the authors and contributors and not of The University of Bristol or The Policy Press. The University of Bristol and The Policy Press disclaim responsibility for any injury to persons or property resulting from any material published in this publication.

The Policy Press works to counter discrimination on grounds of gender, race, disability, age and sexuality.

Cover design by Qube Design Associates, Bristol.
Photograph used kindly supplied by www.johnbirdsall.co.uk.
Printed in Great Britain by Marston Book Services, Oxford.

Executive summary

Research objectives

- The aim of this study was to conduct a longitudinal analysis of the effects of poor housing upon health using data collected as part of the National Child Development Study (NCDS).

- Three research topics were addressed. The first research topic focused on the *link between overcrowding and respiratory and infectious disease*. The second research topic considered *if, and when, housing deprivation impacts upon overall health*. The third research topic entailed *an examination of the link between housing deprivation and health in the context of the range of other possible influences upon health*.

- An important step in addressing the research topics was the construction of appropriate measures for the relevant health and housing variables. In attempting to create appropriate indices for the severity of ill-health and for housing deprivation and subsequently incorporating them into a single analysis this research represents an innovative approach to the analysis of the links between housing and health. Existing studies typically rely on single or simpler indicators which do not always capture the full scope or nature of the phenomena.

Data source

- The NCDS began with a survey of all those born in Great Britain between 3 and 9 March 1958. Subsequent surveys have been conducted in 1965 (age 7), 1969 (age 11), 1974 (age 16),

1981 (age 23) and 1991 (age 33). There are currently plans to conduct a further sweep in 1999. Sweeps 1 and 2 also include people who have immigrated to Great Britain who were born in the relevant time period.

- There were 17,415 respondents to the survey in 1958, which represents some 98% of the relevant cohort. By 1991 the response rate had dropped to 70%, but the representativeness of the cohort was not seriously compromised.

- Perhaps the central concern for policy is whether housing deprivation has an effect upon health independent of the effects of low income. In order to examine this question fully it is desirable to have robust data on income levels. Yet, the information on income which the NCDS offers cannot readily be employed in analysis. Our research relied on the alternative indicators of low income levels which, while less satisfactory than an income measure, none the less allow indicators of low 'standard of living' to enter the analysis.

Key findings

Creating a housing deprivation index

- Our attempt to create a housing deprivation index met with mixed success. The housing deprivation index used drew on a range of NCDS housing variables encompassing physical characteristics, location, satisfaction, past homelessness and independent assessments of housing difficulties. The precise composition of the index varied between sweeps both because the sweeps gathered slightly different data and because the meaning and nature of deprivation changes over time and hence the most appropriate components for a deprivation index need to change if the index is to capture the phenomenon reliably. The variables included in the indices were strongly associated with ill-health, but while the housing-related questions on the NCDS had great relevance in the 1960s their relevance declined rapidly such that for the later sweeps unreliable indices were being generated. The ability of the index to measure housing deprivation accurately was thus considerably lower for later sweeps.

- While the NCDS data displays this feature, it is important to recognise that many of the other indices already in use have similar difficulties and that, in fact, the NCDS performs better than most. None the less, it would be desirable to explore this area further with a more reliable measure of housing deprivation.

Housing pathways

- Attention among epidemiological researchers is increasingly focused upon the way in which health risks of various types – genetic, behavioural, socio-economic – accumulate across the life-course. In this context it is of interest to explore the notion of a 'pathway' of housing conditions from childhood to adulthood. Do people who follow different housing pathways experience different health outcomes?

- Tracing housing pathways over time highlights the apparently diverse housing careers followed by cohort members. Less than a quarter of cohort members never experienced any housing deprivation between birth and age 33, but long-term or repeated experience of multiple housing deprivation was relatively rare (only one in five cohort members experienced multiple deprivation during at least two sweeps).

- Evidence regarding the impact of overcrowding upon respiratory health and infectious disease is mixed. In childhood to age 11 it is associated with a heightened likelihood of experiencing both infectious and respiratory disease while in adulthood it is associated with an increased likelihood of respiratory disease alone. Evidence

regarding the impact of overcrowding upon respiratory health and infectious disease is mixed. In childhood to age 11 it is associated with a heightened likliehood of experiencing both infectious and respiratory disease while in adulthood it is associated with an increased likelihood of respiratory disease alone.

- The association between housing deprivation and more general ill-health indicates that it may play a role in increasing the likelihood of experiencing severe or moderate ill-health in adulthood and early childhood. Our analysis is in accord with much of the existing literature which sees current conditions and, secondly, those existing in childhood as being the most important influences on adult health.

- The evidence provided by our examination of the association between housing pathways and health, without attempting to take other possible health risks into account, does not provide strong support for the proposition that the accumulation of a 'chain' of housing deprivation risks throughout the life-course is a key factor in determining health in adulthood. The evidence from the NCDS could support a number of competing interpretations of the role which housing conditions may play in affecting health outcomes over time.

- The analysis requires broadening to take account of other dimensions of housing deprivation, the accumulation of other types of health risk and the way housing interacts with other health risks in a manner which may result in a 'chain' of risks being formed which results in adverse health outcomes.

Housing in context

- When housing circumstances in adulthood are analysed alongside other current influences upon health, three housing variables – whether the cohort member has been homeless, dissatisfied with the area they live in and living in non-self-contained accommodation (rooms, caravans, etc) – emerge as significant explanatory variables even after controlling for other influences on health.

- From longitudinal analysis addressing the range of factors – social, standard of living, genetic, behavioural – which can affect health, housing deprivation emerges as a very significant explanatory variable even after controlling for the other factors. While the previously mentioned limitations of the data need to be borne in mind, the analysis indicated that the experience of multiple housing deprivation led to a 25% (on average) greater risk of disability or severe ill-health across the life-course of the cohort members in the NCDS.

Housing and health

- Overall, once other factors have been controlled for, housing plays a significant role in health outcomes. The two exhibit a dose–response relationship: greater housing deprivation at one point will lead to a greater probability of ill-health and a sustained experience of housing deprivation over time will increase the probability of ill-health.

- Equally importantly, history matters. Poor current housing conditions in adulthood are associated with greater likelihood of ill-health, but living in non-deprived housing conditions is more likely to be associated with ill-health among those who have experienced housing deprivation earlier in life than among those who have not.

Key implications for policy

- Bearing in mind the issues of the reliability of the housing deprivation index and the absence of a fully satisfactory income measure, the results of the longitudinal analysis suggest that housing deprivation has a substantial effect upon the risk of ill-health. Further work seeking to corroborate and document the biomedical mechanisms involved is desirable, but, when considered in the context of existing research, these results can be seen as indicative of a causal relationship.

- Acting to improve the housing conditions of both adults and children would be of benefit, but addressing the conditions of children in particular would deliver direct benefits in terms of

improved current health and would bring indirect benefits in reducing the likelihood of ill-health in later life.

- Our analysis reinforces existing findings regarding the deleterious effects of homelessness, but in this instance the focus is on the impact of past, rather than current, homelessness upon current health.

- Acting to reduce housing deprivation could therefore have a significant impact upon the nation's health. Among the NCDS cohort, the impact of multiple housing deprivation would appear to be of the same order of magnitude as addressing the issue of smoking and the risk to health posed by multiple housing deprivation seems to be, on average, greater than that posed by excessive alcohol consumption.

- These results have important implications for health policy. Current policy agendas acknowledge housing to be one among a number of influences upon health. Our analysis suggests that, from a longitudinal perspective, this is fully justified and that housing concerns should be an integral and explicit part of health policy. Housing issues and housing policies need to be an integral and important component of thinking and planning. Housing issues and housing organisations need to be given the necessary prominence in planning and resource allocation decisions at the local level if policy initiatives are to bring the greatest benefit to the health of local populations. Current policy at national level appears to have the potential to foster such an approach to health policy: the key question is the extent to which implementation of the current agenda is able to deliver on its potential.

Outstanding methodological issues

- The desirability of a more reliable housing deprivation index implies that there is a need to think about data requirements. A more reliable index requires the collection of data on housing circumstances and conditions which are more appropriate and relevant to British society at the end of the 1990s.

- Further development work on the NCDS in order to ensure that better quality income information were available would be of great value. This would allow the analysis of the NCDS to advance further than has been possible in this study. Without such data, the question as to whether an analysis which could include more accurate income data would lead to modified conclusions remains open.

- Disease contracted in childhood can have effects that only become apparent after a considerable time lag. It may therefore be that the NCDS cohort were not old enough in 1991 for the full import of certain types of infection or respiratory disease experienced in childhood to become apparent. The further sweep of the NCDS to be conducted in 1999 provides an opportunity for any such longer-term consequences to begin to appear.

Introduction

1

Background

The determinants of an individual's health are complex and multifaceted. They include demographic and hereditary factors, individual life-style factors, social and community networks and general socio-economic, cultural and environmental conditions. Housing is one of the key environmental influences upon health. As Blackburn (1990, p 77) notes:

> ... [t]he quality of our home environment has an important bearing on our quality of life. Most people spend at least half of their waking hours at home.... Housing is, therefore, a major health resource.

The link between health and housing conditions is currently moving up the policy agenda in the light of the government's renewed drive to improve the health of the nation. The green paper *Our Healthier Nation* (DoH, 1998) notes health as one of the key environmental factors which affect health. It notes in particular the impact that damp, crowding and cold can have on health. Similarly, the Acheson Report (1998) highlights housing and environment as a key area for future policy development if health inequalities are to lessen. More generally, there is increasing concern with the longer term impacts of poor housing upon health and, consequently, with the implications of poor housing for the demands placed on health and social care services.

In the light of this renewed interest in housing and health in December 1997 the Department of the Environment, Transport and the Regions (DETR) commissioned the research reported here. The research draws on existing secondary data to explore the impact of poor housing upon health.

Scope and objectives

The principal aim of this study was to conduct a longitudinal analysis of the effects of poor housing upon health using data collected as part of the National Child Development Study (NCDS). The NCDS began in 1958 as a Perinatal Mortality Survey (PMS) of all those born in Great Britain between 3-9 March 1958. There have been five subsequent surveys which attempted to trace the cohort members and collect further data. The sweeps were conducted in 1965 (age 7), 1969 (age 11), 1974 (age 16), 1981 (age 23) and 1991 (age 33). There are currently plans to conduct a further sweep in 1999. Sweeps 1 and 2 also include people who have immigrated to Great Britain and who were born in the relevant time period. Table 1 presents the number of cohort members for whom responses are available in each sweep. The sweeps collect very detailed health data for each cohort member, but there is also data covering topics such as the physical, educational and social development of the child cohort members and the employment and life histories of the cohort members as adults. The NCDS therefore represents a substantial and rich potential source of data with which to examine the direct and indirect links between health and housing. More background information on data collection relating to the NCDS can be found in Shepherd (1995) and Appendix E presents a brief analysis of response bias in the NCDS.

Table 1: Response to the sweeps of the NCDS

	Number of responses
Perinatal Mortality Survey (1958)	17,415
Sweep 1 (1965)	15,425
Sweep 2 (1969)	15,337
Sweep 3 (1974)	14,647
Sweep 4 (1981)	12,537
Sweep 5 (1991)	11,407

The first stage of this study examined the literature on the links between housing conditions and health. Particular attention was given to studies which attempted longitudinal analyses of the link. This review made it clear that much of the existing literature examining the impact of housing on health tends either to be cross-sectional or, when attempting to identify the influence of childhood circumstances relative to current circumstances, to take account of childhood and current circumstances without also examining people's experiences and exposure to risk in the intervening period. Yet, it is increasingly recognised by epidemiological researchers that this approach is not sufficient.

Attention is increasingly being focused upon the way in which health risks of various types – genetic, behavioural, socio-economic – are accumulated across the life-course. Do risks accumulate across the life-course to form 'links in a chain' leading to adverse health outcomes? If so, does breaking the chain prevent early health risks translating into adverse health outcomes? In this context it is of interest to explore the notion of a 'pathway' from childhood to adulthood. Do people who follow different pathways – both housing and non-housing – experience different health outcomes, either contemporaneous and/or cumulative?

While the analysis of health risk over the life-course has only recently begun to attract attention, it is equally clear that where attempts have been made to incorporate housing deprivation into analyses of socio-economic influences upon health it has been treated relatively crudely. The small amount of literature which considers housing issues has often drawn on the NCDS. Not only has the consideration of housing often been relatively crude, but explicit consideration of housing deprivation has not featured in much of the existing literature.

Instead there is a reliance upon more general measures of socio-economic conditions. There is therefore considerable scope for examining the possibility of deriving more sophisticated indicators of housing deprivation for use in the analysis of the impact of housing upon health.

The second stage of this study involved the analysis of the NCDS and addressed research topics in three broad areas. The first topic focused on the link between overcrowding and respiratory health and infectious disease. More specifically, we sought to examine the following questions:

- How are different pathways of overcrowding associated with respiratory disease?
- Are subjects who experience overcrowding in childhood more likely to suffer respiratory disease in childhood and/or later life?
- Are subjects who experience overcrowding in childhood prone to respiratory disease throughout life or does it (re)emerge at a later stage in life?
- Are subjects who experience overcrowding more likely to suffer infectious disease?
- If overcrowding increases the likelihood of suffering infectious disease, is this effect tied to current housing conditions or does it persist once overcrowding is reduced?

The second topic considered if, and when, housing deprivation impacts upon overall health. It sought to examine the following questions:

- How does the experience of housing deprivation impact upon ill-health?
- How does the timing and duration of housing deprivation differ between subjects and does the experience of ill-health at different points in development and for differing durations have differing impacts upon health?

Finally an examination of the link between housing deprivation and health in the context of the range of other possible influences upon health was undertaken by means of a longitudinal analysis on the basis of a life-course perspective on health risks. This third topic sought to examine the following questions:

- What effect does the experience of housing deprivation at different points in the life-course have upon health, once the range of other influences upon quality of health are incorporated into the analysis?
- Does the NCDS provide any evidence that housing deprivation has indirect and long-term effects upon health?
- Is there any evidence that good housing acts as a 'protective factor' for those exposed to other health risks?

An important step in addressing the research topics was the construction of appropriate measures for the relevant health and housing variables. In attempting to operationalise appropriate indices this study represents an innovative approach to the analysis of the links between housing and health. Existing studies typically rely on simpler indicators which do not always capture the full scope of the phenomena under investigation. The data available on the NCDS allowed considerable progress towards the use of more sophisticated indicators of both housing deprivation and health, but the attempt to create a housing deprivation index raised important questions about the appropriate methods for measuring housing deprivation in the 1990s and beyond. While the analysis produced some valuable findings, the nature of the available data means that the housing deprivation measure which underpins the analysis was not as robust as might have been desirable.

Structure of the report

Chapter 2 of this report presents the key findings from the existing literature on health, housing and socio-economic conditions and considers the rationale for a life-course or pathways approach to the analysis of health. An important stepping stone in addressing the research topics outlined above is the construction of appropriate measures for the relevant health variables. Our approach is described in Chapter 3.

Chapters 4, 5 and 6 present the results of our analysis of the NCDS. Chapter 4 focuses upon the link between overcrowded accommodation and the experience of respiratory and infectious disease. At the start of Chapter 5 we present an explanation of

the thinking behind the construction of housing deprivation measures and then present a summary of our analysis of housing deprivation using the NCDS data. This chapter then goes on to explore the link between this measure of housing deprivation and the severity of ill-health experienced by the NCDS cohort members. Our longitudinal analysis of the NCDS is presented in Chapter 6. The main task of this chapter is to attempt to disentangle the effects of housing deprivation upon health, allowing for the influence of a range of other possible causal factors. The final chapter briefly summarises the key messages to emerge from the research. It presents some of the policy implications that flow from the results of the research.

2

What do we know about the influence of housing on health?

The effects of poor housing on health have been recognised in the scientific literature for over 150 years, since Chadwick (1842) estimated the average life expectancy of people in Liverpool in the worst housing (cellars) to be only 15 years. While the relationship between housing conditions and physical and psychological health has been a recurrent topic for scientific investigation, the nature of the relationship between health-related outcomes and current housing quality and housing history has only relatively recently begun to be understood. Sonja Hunt (1997), writing in the recent Registrar General Decennial Supplement, noted that "there has been surprisingly little scientific research on housing and health" (pp 161-2). More specifically, we can distinguish three different ways in which housing enters into analyses of the determinants of health. Firstly, there is a relatively large amount of literature on inequalities in health that utilises housing tenure as a classificatory variable. Secondly, cross-sectional studies link various 'poor' current housing conditions with current ill-health. Thirdly, there is a relatively small amount of literature which attempts to explore the longitudinal effects of 'poor' housing conditions on ill-health. Current housing conditions have been found to impact upon various dimensions of health, but our principle concern in this chapter is with the third branch of the existing literature. We seek to review the evidence on the long-term impact of housing conditions on health drawn from longitudinal studies. Key concerns are the direct and indirect effects that a poor housing environment at an early stage in the life cycle may have upon health in later life.

Before moving on to consider the findings from this literature we note that while the literature which examines the link between health outcomes and housing is relatively small there is a larger amount of literature which examines the links between health and measures of socio-economic circumstances other than housing. We do not review this literature here but simply note that where studies rely on single or simple measures of socio-economic circumstances, these measures may be acting as a proxy for a number of different health risks, some of which may have an unexplored housing dimension.

The main body of this chapter is in six parts. We first examine the range of possible links between housing and health in order to clarify the scope of the current study. We then examine very briefly the results of the cross-sectional literature before focusing on longitudinal questions. We end by considering the emergence of life-course approaches to the understanding of health which, we suggest, represent a significant advance upon previous approaches: one which has considerable potential to enhance and advance our understanding of the long-term impacts of housing circumstances on health.

Linking health and housing

At one level the link between poor housing environments and poor health has been taken to be self-evident: many of the early interventions in public health were directed at addressing poor housing conditions in the belief that this would improve the health of the nation. The improvements in health subsequent to these interventions provides, at the very least, circumstantial evidence that this belief was well founded, even if the precise mechanisms by which improved housing resulted in better health were not always well understood.

At an analytical level, it has proved much harder to demonstrate beyond dispute the nature and magnitude of the effect that housing conditions have upon health. There are a number of possible ways in which housing and health could be linked:

- A poor current housing environment could impact directly upon the health of residents.

- A poor housing environment at an early stage in the life cycle may have a direct and adverse effect upon health in later life, even when in later life an individual's housing circumstances cease to be poor.

- Poor housing in childhood which results in poor health may mean that children do not fully develop physically and socially and therefore do not realise their potential through education. This in turn means that the individual occupies a less favourable socio-economic position in adulthood than would otherwise be the case. This in turn carries with it health implications.

- Good quality housing may act as a protective factor against the effect of other socio-economic disadvantages.

- Access to housing may be conditional upon health such that, for example, those with poor health tend to be allocated to particular parts of the housing system by either their reduced ability to access the labour market or their increased eligibility to access administratively allocated housing.

Each of these possibilities is plausible, but there are a number of analytical difficulties to be overcome. On the one hand, poor housing conditions are frequently encountered alongside other indicators of social disadvantage and it can be difficult to isolate the independent effect of poor housing upon health. On the other hand, it may be that the effects of poor housing on health may be indirect and take a number of years to manifest themselves. In order to isolate such effects it is therefore necessary to disentangle the effect of housing from a whole range of confounding factors. Approaching the problem from the other direction, it is possible that good quality housing can act as a protective factor against other socio-economic disadvantages, but here again in order to identify such an effect it

is necessary to control for a wide range of possible confounding factors.

The difficulty in identifying the independent effect of housing on health has led some to call for the use of an holistic method (eg Thunhurst, 1993) which accepts some ambiguity regarding the identification of causation. The alternative view is that analysis needs to be approached with greater sophistication and an appreciation of the need for greater diligence and precision in accounting for the effects of confounding variables (Davey Smith and Phillips, 1992).

The question as to whether health selection operates within the housing market has been examined by Smith and colleagues (Smith, 1990; Smith and Mallinson, 1997a, 1997b) and Robinson (1998) has recently extended the analysis to incorporate the impact of homelessness upon subsequent housing position. We do not consider this issue in detail.

The impact of current housing on health

The literature on current housing conditions and health points to the conclusion that current housing can have significant impacts upon health. This literature has been reviewed extensively by a number of authors (eg Smith, 1989; Lowry, 1991; Arblaster and Hawtin, 1993; Ineichen, 1993; Leather et al, 1994; Universities of Sussex and Westminster, 1996; Hunt, 1997). In seeking to examine the longer-term impacts of housing upon health, current housing conditions are an important confounding factor which need to be taken into account if any independent effect of housing history is to be identified.

For current purposes it is sufficient to note that 'poor' current housing can impact upon both physical and mental health and that the aspects of poor housing which impact upon current health vary, to some extent, with stages of the life cycle. Particular types of housing disadvantage have a greater effect upon children and child development than upon adult health, while some represent problems particularly for older people. Tables 2 and 3 draw primarily upon the discussion by Hunt (1997) to summarise the key messages from the cross-sectional literature.

Table 2: The consequences of 'poor' housing circumstance for physical health

Housing circumstance	Consequence	Relevant studies
Overcrowding	– increased risk of infectious or respiratory disease – reduced stature	Montgomery et al (1996); Hunt et al (1997)
Damp and mould	– respiratory problems eg wheeze – asthma, rhinitis and alveolitis – eczema	Strachan and Elton (1986); Platt-Mills and Chapman (1987); Burr et al (1988); Platt et al (1989); Hyndman (1990); Dales et al (1991); Dekker et al (1991); Miller (1992); Sporik et al (1992); Packer et al (1994); Spengler et al (1994); Verhoeff et al (1995); Hopton and Hunt (1996); Williamson et al (1997)
Indoor pollutants and infestation	– asthma	Weitzman et al (1990); Chapman (1993); Rona and Chinn (1993); Cook and Strachan (1997); Ashmore (1998)
Cold	– diminished resistance to respiratory infection – hypothermia – bronchospasm – ischaemic heart disease, myocardial infarction and strokes	Collins (1986); Blackman et al (1989); Strachan and Sanders (1989); Collins (1993)
Homelessness – rooflessness	– problems resulting from facing the elements without protection	Shanks and Smith (1992); Bines (1997)
Homelessness – temporary accommodation	– problems resulting from overcrowding, noise, inadequate cooking and washing facilities	Conway (1988, 1993)

Table 3: The consequences of 'poor' housing circumstance for mental health

Housing circumstance	Consequence	Relevant studies
Relatively poor quality housing in each tenure	– residents' mental well-being reduced	Platt et al (1989); Hunt (1990); Payne (1991); Hopton and Hunt (1996); Payne (1997)
'Difficult-to-let' housing	– poorer emotional well-being than people in 'better' areas	Blackman et al (1989)
Damp	– depression in women	Brown and Harris (1978); Hyndman (1990)
Overcrowding	– results in emotional problems, developmental delay and bed-wetting, poorer educational attainment and mental adjustment in children – social tension, irritability, impairment of social relations	Murray (1974); Rutter (1974); Arblaster (1994); Montgomery et al (1996); Hunt (1997)
Flatted accommodation	– increased GP consultation by women for emotional symptoms – social isolation and psychiatric disturbance among women	Fanning (1967); Stewart (1970); Ineichen and Hooper (1974); Freeman (1993); Gabe and Williams (1993)

Health and poor socio-economic circumstances in childhood: the link with adulthood

A range of evidence exists to indicate that the quality of health experienced by children is directly related to their socio-economic position. Living in disadvantaged socio-economic circumstances is associated with relatively poor health (see, for example, Bor et al, 1993) and that, when subject to the same health injuries, those from deprived backgrounds suffered greater ill-effects (Wyke et al, 1991). Reading (1997), for example, has recently reviewed the literature which examines the association between social disadvantage and infection in childhood. His review indicates that, while some infections exhibit no social gradient to childhood infection and for others the evidence of a social gradient is equivocal, there is considerable evidence that many types of infectious disease – including respiratory diseases, gastroenteritis, *Helicobacter pylori* infection and tuberculosis – exhibit a strong social gradient in childhood.

The question of most concern for this study is whether these findings regarding childhood are of significance for the analysis of health outcomes in adulthood. Specifically, is such childhood ill-health caused by housing? Do they carry with them longer-term implications for health in later life? With reference to the first of these questions, the studies reported in Table 2 suggest that poor housing environments are a factor in the experience of at least some of these diseases. With regard to the second question, Power and Peckham (1990), for example, drew on the NCDS to examine morbidity in childhood and adult ill-health. They concluded that the state of health in childhood had long-term implications but that it did not make a substantial contribution to ill-health in early adulthood (see also Power et al, 1991). Martyn (1991), on the other hand, argues that for pulmonary infections there is evidence that infection in childhood can lead to persisting abnormalities of lung function which may have permanent deleterious effects. Similarly, chronic exposure to fungal spores resulting from dampness may lead to irreversible changes in lung function (Tobin et al, 1987). Fuller understanding of these issues can only be gained by considering housing and socio-economic conditions in the context of other health risks and in an explicitly longitudinal framework.

The impact of past housing conditions on health

We turn now to studies which attempt, with greater or lesser sophistication, to take account of housing history in examining determinants of current health.

Housing in childhood and health

The most frequently employed indicator of housing conditions is overcrowding. A study by Brittan et al (1987) found that overcrowding (more than 2 persons per room) at the age of two was one of only four significant explanatory variables in their analysis of respiratory problems in 36-year-old men and women. Barker et al (1990) found an association between domestic crowding in early life and stomach cancer. Short stature in adulthood, which is a risk factor for a number of diseases including heart disease, has also been found to be associated with overcrowding in earlier life (Kuh and Wadsworth, 1989). In contrast, Coggon et al (1993) found little evidence that the housing of young adults in the 1930s had an effect upon their later mortality from a range of diseases including stomach cancer and rheumatic heart disease.

Mendall et al (1992) considered both domestic crowding and absence of a fixed hot water supply at age 8 in their study of *Helicobacter pylori* seropositivity in adult life. They found that after controlling for age, sex, current social class and the number of children in the current household, *crowding* and the presence of hot water in childhood were powerful independent risk factors for current infection with *Helicobacter pylori*.

Using the Medical Research Council (MRC) National Survey of Health and Development, Mann et al (1992) investigated the factors influencing respiratory illness. They found that for those born in 1946 poor home environment (defined as lacking amenities and overcrowding), parental bronchitis, atmospheric pollution, childhood lower respiratory tract illness and later smoking were the best predictors of adult lower respiratory tract illness.

They concluded that the accumulation of risk in childhood and adolescence had significant implications for later adult problems.

Housing during early life and health

A small number of studies have employed the NCDS to analyse the impact of housing upon health longitudinally. Ghodsian and Fogelman (1988) used the first four sweeps of the NCDS to look at the impact of housing and social circumstances on a range of outcomes, including health. They found that, allowing for the sex of subject, self-rated health at age 23 was statistically significantly related to tenure, where tenure was dichotomised (owner/renter) and subjects were allocated to one of four groups according to tenure at ages 7, 11, and 16 (owner throughout, renter throughout, tenant to owner, and owner to tenant). Those in owner-occupation throughout were more likely to rate their health excellent/good than others, particularly those who had moved from owner-occupation to renting during childhood.

Type of accommodation in childhood was not significantly related to self-rated health, but both the subject's experience of crowding and lack of amenities were. Allowing for subject's sex and their parents' education, those not crowded at any time were the most likely to rate their health as excellent/good at age 23. Such subjects were 1.6 times more likely to consider their health excellent/ good than those who had been crowded throughout childhood or crowded at age 7 but not at 16. Those who only moved to crowded accommodation later in childhood showed little difference in their likelihood of rating their health excellent/good.

Ghodsian and Fogelman's (1988) results relating to amenities incorporate an interaction between amenities and neighbourhood. The variables which enter their model are sex, parents' education, neighbourhood, and the interaction between neighbourhood and amenities. They concluded that contrasts in self-rated health at age 23 associated with differing levels of amenities in childhood varied according to the type of neighbourhood the subject grew up in.

The most dramatic contrast in health rating is between those that grew up in the best off neighbourhoods and those from 'deprived' or 'other' neighbourhoods. The broad picture was of those who grew up with good amenities being most likely to rate their health highly, although the differences are not great among those from 'deprived' or 'other' neighbourhoods. Within the best off areas, though, there was a much greater difference between those with good amenities during childhood and those without. On the basis of this data, Ghodsian and Fogelman argue that "It is reasonable to conclude that the disadvantages for subsequent feelings about one's health associated with having grown up with inadequate amenities appear to be greater if experienced in the contrasting setting of a well off neighbourhood" (1988, p 75). This suggests an important subjective and relative component to housing deprivation.

Their study also examined the impact of housing in childhood upon the malaise score, which is designed to detect the likelihood of being depressed. They found that high malaise scores (which indicate a greater likelihood of being depressed) occurred least frequently among subjects who had been in owner-occupation throughout childhood and among those who lived in whole houses throughout their childhood. Those who were crowded throughout childhood exhibited the highest malaise scores at age 23.

Power (1991) also used data from the first four sweeps of the NCDS to examine how controlling for early socio-economic background modifies the impact of social class on four measures of health (self-rated health, 'malaise', psychological morbidity and height). She found that housing tenure and crowding in earlier life, along with family size and receipt of free school meals, substantially reduced the class differentials in health. Alongside these factors, more recent unemployment and family formation were also important.

Power et al (1991) elaborated on this work by incorporating aspects of individual health behaviour, inheritance at birth, and childhood illness alongside housing and other socio-economic indicators. They reiterated that more recent socio-economic circumstances – specifically recent unemployment (for men) and family formation (for women) –

appeared more important in determining health than earlier circumstances. The authors conducted a multivariate analysis using indicators from each of the broad areas which have been identified as possible determinants of health (for example, socio-economic circumstances, health behaviour, etc). They concluded that the indicators of socio-economic background (social class at birth and housing tenure at age 11), which they separated into earlier and later circumstances, were especially relevant to psychological morbidity in men and self-rated health and malaise in women. They observed that some of the effect of the socio-economic variables which was apparent in bivariate analysis was reduced once adjustments were made for variables representing other areas.

Moving to a life-course approach to the analysis of health

Controlling for current socio-economic circumstances is essential if the independent effect of childhood circumstances is to be identified. Yet, researchers are increasingly recognising that analysis needs to move beyond this dichotomy (current/childhood) to examine how socio-economic circumstances over the life-course affect the accumulation of health risk and the experience of poor health in adulthood. Increased attention is therefore being directed at life-course approaches to epidemiology which propose an explanatory framework which can encompass the range of biological, behavioural and socio-economic factors from heredity and fetal growth, through childhood and on into adulthood (Kuh and Ben-Shlomo, 1997).

Power and Hertzman (1997) made a number of pertinent observations. They noted that many epidemiological investigations emphasise the independence of the risks associated with a particular factor such as poor housing environments at particular stages in the life-course. In contrast, they suggested that an approach which might be more useful is one which tries "to understand how risks experienced at different ages *combine* to increase risk of disease in adult life" (1997, p 215, emphasis as original). This would allow a more accurate representation of the complex relationships between social and biological influences upon

health across the life-course. Such a conceptualisation might hypothesise that there are a number of intervening 'links in the chain' which are required before illness follows as the long-term consequences of a particular health risk. If some of those links are absent then the later illness may not occur. Power and Hertzman observed that some early life insults can be altered in ways which affect subsequent risk of disease. They noted that it is not known which such insults cannot be ameliorated at a later stage. Nor have the adult diseases for which early life factors are more important than later factors been identified with any great certainty.

An earlier paper by West (1988) observed health gradients across social classes in childhood which equalised in youth, only to reappear in young adulthood. This suggests that the simple proposition that those in lower socio-economic groups face worse socio-economic circumstances throughout life and hence experience relatively poor health throughout life is not sustainable. The mechanisms involved in generating health inequalities may be more complex and indirect than is frequently assumed.

The alternative conception proposed by Power and Hertzman offers a suggestive framework for exploring these issues. It could move research away from studies which simply correlate, for example, housing conditions in childhood with later adult illness while, possibly, controlling for current circumstances and towards research which traces pathways from childhood to adulthood and provides plausible accounts of the links in the chain between the two. Such research would be truly longitudinal. Data to undertake this type of work is rarely available, but the NCDS offers a valuable resource with which to explore the possibilities.

Although life-course approaches have not yet been extensively explored empirically, studies are emerging which indicate the relevant issues. The housing dimension to these issues has yet, however, to be fully examined.

Power et al (1996) used the NCDS to tackle the health selection argument (Blane et al, 1993; Fox et al, 1985) by addressing the question of whether lifetime social circumstances or social mobility determine health inequalities. Their outcome measures are drawn from sweep 5 of the NCDS. They concluded that, contrary to the health selection argument, lifetime socio-economic circumstances rather than social mobility are the major influence on health inequalities (see also Davey Smith et al, 1997). This work is extended by Power et al (1997) who examined whether social gradients for specific health problems had changed for the NCDS cohort members between sweeps 4 and 5. They concluded that while inequalities did not appear to widen, this varied across health measures. The implication is that inequalities may reproduce through different pathways, only some of which may be related to socio-economic position.

More recently Power and Matthews (1997) used the five sweeps of the NCDS to examine the origins of health inequalities. They were particularly concerned as to whether risks accumulated differentially by social position over the life-course. The authors examined the range of health risks under the following headings: economic circumstances, health-related behaviour, social and family functioning and structure and educational achievement and work career. The authors included the following housing factors: overcrowding, lacking or sharing household amenities, renting housing (age 33) and problems with paying for housing. They concluded that an individual's chance of encountering multiple adverse health risks throughout life was influenced powerfully by social position. The social trends which are observed in adult disease risk factors accumulate over decades, rather than emerging exclusively in mid-life. The paper does not, however, bring the various risks together into a multivariate analysis.

Summary

There are a number of plausible ways in which housing and health could be related. The literature indicates that a number of dimensions of current housing circumstances can impact upon health, particularly in relation to respiratory problems. That the housing circumstances of children can cause serious ill-health is of particular concern in the light of the evidence that such ill-health can cause damage which carries through into adulthood, although the strength of this long-term effect is by no means established with any certainty.

In the analysis of health outcomes in adulthood current housing is a confounding factor to be controlled for in order to explore the role of past housing. Attempts to examine current and past housing circumstances together point to housing history having an impact. Some authors find that housing in childhood emerges strongly as a factor associated with particular types of adult disease, while others argue that past housing has an effect on adult health but that this effect is dominated by the impact of current circumstances and behaviours.

The move away from a simple distinction between childhood and current circumstances represents an important development in the understanding of health outcomes in adulthood. It points to the need to examine the accumulation of the full range – socio-economic, behavioural, social, etc – of risks throughout the life-course in order to see how such risks can reinforce or interact with each other to generate particular health outcomes. People in different social classes are likely to experience different housing-related risks; whether such risks form links in a 'housing risk chain' which itself results in adverse health outcomes in adulthood or are part of some larger accumulation of risk is still to be explored.

3

Measuring health: the construction of the health measures used in this study

Before analysing the effects of housing conditions upon health it is necessary to construct suitable measures for the various dimensions of health we are interested in. This section describes the thinking behind the measures constructed and details the components that went into each measure. These measures are used in the remainder of this report.

Infectious and respiratory disease

In order to address the objectives of the first research topic one it was necessary to construct measures for both infectious and respiratory disease. The sweeps of the NCDS collect information on a range of infectious and respiratory disease which the subjects may have experienced. The information collected at different times varied somewhat. The most important differences are that at age 7 the information related to whether the subject had experienced a particular disease/illness at any point in their life, while the subsequent two sweeps focused on the experience of disease either ever, since the last sweep, in the preceding year or the age the cohort member was when a disease/illness was first experienced. The sweeps also differed in the measures used to indicate a cohort member had experienced a disease. In the early sweeps the indicator was a report by the cohort member's mother that the cohort member had experienced the disease/illness and this included, at the age of 16, absence from school or visits to the GP for the condition. At age 23 the main concern was long-standing illness, reasons for hospital admissions or regular medical supervision. At age 33 long-standing illness was sub-divided into limiting or non-limiting long-standing illness and reasons for

hospital admissions and the receipt of medical supervision were also considered.

The range of infectious diseases which the NCDS subjects could have experienced is clearly considerable and the survey, in the early years in particular, restricted itself to the most common. The fact that some of these diseases are so common is a methodological issue in the current study. During this century there has been a dramatic reduction in morbidity and mortality from the common infectious childhood diseases of measles, mumps, chickenpox and rubella. Harvey and Kovar (1985) argue that this is the product of improved housing conditions, better sanitation and nutrition, and the introduction of vaccines.

However, the NCDS cohort members would have been expected to experience the four common infectious childhood diseases during their childhood. Only 5% of individuals in the population reached adulthood without catching chickenpox, with the attack rate among non-immune households being greater than 90% (Southgate et al, 1997). Measles notifications reached half a million in the 1960s (Donaldson and Donaldson, 1983) when it was essentially universal in the UK. Rubella too, was endemic in Britain, with periodic epidemics in children. Mumps epidemics tended to occur in four yearly cycles (for example, 1970/71, 1974/75, 1978) but their size has lessened since the mumps vaccine was first introduced in the 1950s (Donaldson and Donaldson, 1983).

In the light of the high incidence of the four common infectious childhood diseases – measles, mumps, chickenpox and rubella – while the NCDS cohort members were growing up, a summary measure for infectious disease which included them would be extremely insensitive to variations in socio-economic conditions or any other potential causal factor. It was therefore decided that they should be excluded from the measure of infectious disease used in this study in order that we could focus upon the link between housing conditions and a more specific range of less frequently occurring infectious diseases. The diseases which we included in our measure of infectious disease at each sweep of the NCDS are presented in Table 4. The list includes the major airborne infections which are usually spread by close contact (Mood, 1993).

For each sweep, dichotomous variables representing experienced illness/not experienced illness were created for both respiratory illness and infectious disease. Each cohort member for whom the relevant data were available was allocated to a category on each variable. Thus, each cohort member recorded up to six observations with regard to respiratory illness and up to six with regard to infectious disease.

It is important to note that as a result of the introduction of the MMR (measles, mumps and rubella) vaccine in 1988 the almost universal childhood experience of a number of infectious diseases among the NCDS cohort would not be replicated today. If we were conducting our analysis of children growing up in contemporary society these diseases would probably be included in a measure of infectious disease, with the likely exception of chickenpox, although the pattern of illness would, in part at least, reflect the uptake of vaccination rather than disadvantaged circumstances per se.

Table 4 also details the components of the measure of respiratory disease that we employ in the study. As can be seen, in childhood the measure focuses upon whether the subject has experienced pneumonia or suffers from asthma, bronchitis with wheezing, or an abnormal respiratory system. Once the subjects reach adulthood the measure broadens to include, for example, chronic obstructive pulmonary disease, pneumoconioses and other lung diseases due to external agents.

An index of the severity of ill-health

The second topic is to consider if, and when, housing deprivation impacts upon overall health, while the last research topic entails an examination of the link between housing deprivation and health in the context of the range of other possible influences upon health. Central to exploring these research topics is the derivation of a summary measure for the severity of ill-health experienced by the NCDS cohort members. Although such summary measures have been proposed in the past, the existing literature has made very little use of them. We believe that this study therefore represents a novel approach to the issue.

For a number of reasons, mortality statistics are widely used as a (rather perverse) indicator of health, because of their availability and reliability and the difficulties of using alternative measures. However, there are a number of indicators of morbidity which may be regarded as more closely aligned to the health–ill-health spectrum. 'Official' morbidity statistics, more commonly collected for administrative or public health use, are of limited use: for example, the rate of absence from work depends upon access to the labour market, or the rate of contact with the health service depends upon the service supply and referral practices. Thus, these and a number of more ad hoc measures have been adopted in this study to provide an estimate of health measurement.

Blaxter (1989) identified three different models that may be adopted to measure morbidity (Table 5), derived empirically from an analysis of survey questions used in a wide range of European countries.

Table 4: Definition of health measures for infectious and respiratory disease

Sweep	Variable	Definition
1958: birth	Respiratory	Non-specific respiratory disease
	Infectious	Non-specific infectious disease
1965: age 7	Respiratory	Ever had asthma attack; *or* bronchitis with wheezing; *or* pneumonia; *or* has abnormal respiratory system
	Infectious	Ever had whooping cough; *or* scarlet fever; *or* glandular fever/tuberculosis
1969: age 11	Respiratory	Has had asthma, wheezing bronchitis between the ages of 7 and 11; *or* has had prescriptions because of wheezing; *or* has been absent from school as a result of bronchitis or asthma
	Infectious *or* meningitis; *or* tuberculosis	Ever had whooping cough; *or* scarlet fever; *or* rheumatic fever; *or* infectious hepatitis;
1974: age 16	Respiratory	Has been absent from school as a result of bronchitis, or asthma/wheezing for one week in the last year; *or* has attended the GP for asthma/wheezing in the last year; *or* suffers from disability relating to asthma or some other chest condition; *or* has suffered from asthma, wheezing or bronchitis since the age of 7
	Infectious	Has been absent from school as a result of a non-specific infectious disease; *or* has attended the GP for infectious fever, gastroenteritis or some other infectious disease in the last year
1981: age 23	Respiratory	Respondent's disability *or* supervised condition *or* hospital admission related to: acute respiratory infections; other diseases of upper respiratory tract; pneumonia; chronic obstructive pulmonary disease and allied conditions; pneumoconioses and other lung diseases due to external agents or other diseases of the respiratory system *or* whether the respondent has suffered from asthma or bronchitis in the last 12 months *or* has had prescribed medicines for asthma or bronchitis in the last 12 months *or* respondent is receiving medical supervision for asthma or bronchitis *or* whether respondent coughs first thing in the morning *or* whether respondent coughs first thing in the morning in winter *or* whether respondent coughs during the day or night *or* whether the respondent coughs up phlegm first thing in the morning in winter *or* whether respondent brings up phlegm during day or night in winter
	Infectious	Respondent's disability *or* supervised condition *or* most recent hospital admission related to: intestinal infectious diseases; tuberculosis; zootonic bacterial diseases; other bacterial diseases; poliomyelitis and other non-arthropod-borne viral diseases of the central nervous system; viral diseases accompanied by exanthem; arthropod-borne viral diseases; other diseases due to viruses and Chalamydiae; rickettsioses and other arthropod-borne diseases; syphilis and other venereal diseases; other spirochaetal; mycoses; helminthiases; other infectious and parasitic diseases; and late effects of infectious and parasitic diseases
1991: age 33	Respiratory	Respondent's long-standing illness or most recent hospital admission related to: acute respiratory infections; other diseases of upper respiratory tract; pneumonia; chronic obstructive pulmonary disease and allied conditions; pneumoconioses and other lung diseases due to external agents or other diseases of respiratory system *or* whether the respondent has ever suffered bronchitis in the last year, *or* whether respondent has seen the doctor in the last year as a result of suffering from bronchitis *or* whether respondent usually coughs first thing in the morning *or* whether respondent usually coughs during the day or night *or* whether the respondent has been coughing most days for three last three months, *or* whether the respondent usually brings up phlegm first thing in the morning *or* whether the respondent brings up phlegm during the day
	Infectious	Respondent's long-standing illness or most recent hospital admission related to: intestinal infectious diseases; tuberculosis; zootonic bacterial diseases; other bacterial diseases; poliomyelitis and other non-arthropod-borne viral diseases of the central nervous system; viral diseases accompanied by exanthem; arthropod-borne viral diseases; other diseases due to viruses and Chalamydiae; rickettsioses and other arthropod-borne diseases; syphilis and other venereal diseases; other spirochaetal; mycoses; helminthiases; other infectious and parasitic diseases; and late effects of infectious and parasitic diseases

Table 5: Different models for measuring morbidity

Medical or physiological/ psychiatric model	Social-interactional or functional model	Subjective or 'illness' model
Clinical examination, physiological/psychiatric screening for abnormality	Tests of physical or psychological disability	Self-assessment of health
and/or	*and/or*	*and/or*
Medical diagnosis of physical or psychiatric disease	Ascertainment of functional status associated with ill-health	Reported experience of physical symptoms of ill-health
and/or	*and/or*	*and/or*
Self-reports of the existence of medically defined disease or abnormality	Inability to perform 'normal' tasks because of disease, impairment or illness	Reported experience of psychosocial malaise

Source: Blaxter (1989)

For obvious reasons, this study has not restricted itself to the wholesale adoption of just one model. For example, there is little or no *self*-reported (as opposed to that reported by parents/carers) information about health in the Perinatal Mortality Survey (PMS), nor in sweeps 1 or 2 of the NCDS, when the cohort members were aged 7 and 11. In contrast, a clinical examination of the cohort members was not undertaken in sweeps 4 or 5 of the NCDS, when the cohort members were aged 23 and 33. Thus, the health measure items selected in this study are, in general, taken from the first two of the three Blaxter models during the childhood of the cohort members and from the last two of her models during the adulthood of the cohort members. It must therefore be borne in mind that the health measures constructed for use at birth and the ages of 7, 11 and 16 represent a more conventional interpretation of the concept of disease, while those constructed for use at the ages of 23 and 33 represent a more conventional interpretation of the concept of illness.

The final items used and the categorisations of health measures used in this study, are, inevitably, to some extent, open to debate. Some inspiration has been provided by the NCDS-related studies on morbidity by Power and Peckham (1988) and Blaxter (1986), and from the thresholds of disability adopted by the Office of Population Censuses and Surveys (OPCS) Surveys of Disability in Great Britain (Bone and Meltzer, 1989). The availability of data at each sweep in the NCDS has naturally been of considerable importance. It must therefore be recognised that the health measures constructed

for the purposes of this study cannot be seen as the definitive answer to the question as to how to measure morbidity; rather they provide a guideline.

The first stage in constructing the health measures was to focus on a number of variables that could be incorporated into specific morbidity groupings. These groupings were of cohort members reported to have: chronic medical problems; chronic physical problems; chronic sensory problems; asthma/bronchitis or wheezing problems; psychosocial problems; psychosomatic problems; and allergies. The second stage in constructing the health measures was to then devise a four-stage index ranging from 'disability/severe health problems' at Scale 1 to 'no health problems' at Scale 4, using a successive filtering process. These scales or 'health measures' were constructed for each of the five sweeps of the NCDS. A summary of the items included in each scale of each measure are given in Table 6 (see also Appendix A for further details). It is important to be clear regarding the status of 'disability' within this framework because it may not be immediately evident that any link between housing conditions and health extends to disability.

Table 7 presents the internationally agreed World Health Organisation (WHO) definition of impairment, disability and handicap in the International Classification of Impairments, Disabilities and Handicaps (ICIDH). Disability is defined as the effects of an impairment on a person's ability to perform activities. How much an impairment affects a person's activities is crucially dependent on their environment, and in particular on their housing environment. The latest revision

Table 6: Summary of the items included in each scale of each 'health measure'

| Health status | Indicators | |
	Childhood	Adulthood
'Disabled/severe health problem'	• in special education • moderate/severe physical handicap or disability • epileptic fit in last year • lacks normal bowel control	• registered disabled • limiting long-standing illness, disability or infirmity • epileptic fit in last year • permanent economic inactivity because of sickness or disability • receipt of Invalidity Benefit, attendance or mobility allowance
'Moderate health problem' (if not already included in above group)	• chronic physical, medical or sensory conditions, asthma or psychosocial problems • slight handicap, hearing or visual problems • more than one month off school in last year	• non-limiting long-standing illness, disability or infirmity • any regular medical supervision • medical supervision for particular conditions such as epilepsy or high blood pressure • two or more hospital admissions in last year • specialist seen for psychiatric • describes own health as poor problems
'Some health problems' (if not already included in above group)	• allergic or psychomatic condition(s) some (non-handicapping) medical condition • hospital admission/outpatient • recent bone fracture	• cough/phlegm in winter • consulted medical practitioner about named condition within last year • hospital admission in last year • work absence because of back pain • describes health as 'not so good'
'No health problems'	All other cohort members	All other cohort members

Table 7: Concepts of 'disablement' used in the ICIDH

Impairment:	any loss or abnormality of psychological, physiological or anatomical structure or function.
Disability:	any restriction or lack (resulting from an impairment) of ability to perform an activity in the manner or within the range considered normal for a human being.
Handicap:	a disadvantage for a given individual, resulting from an impairment or disability, that limits or prevents the fulfillment of a role (depending on age, sex, as well as upon social and cultural factors) for that individual.

of the ICIDH (ICIDH-2 Beta-1 field trials, June 1997) recognises this. The WHO assumption that 'poor' housing conditions may be causally related to disability is also supported by the Department of Health and the Office for National Statistics. The approach we adopt is thus widely accepted.

Comparing the health measures with those from other sources

The final stage of the construction of the measures consisted of attempting to compare the proportions within each measure with other health/disability surveys in order to gauge their accuracy. However, the scope for such comparisons is limited for two broad reasons. Firstly, as already mentioned, the task of quantifying disability in particular is difficult because disability may be regarded as a social construct and definitions will be inevitably contested. Abberley (1996, p 182) comments that the statistics produced by health/disability surveys depend on the "interests, intentions and unexamined presuppositions of those with the power to define and the ability of those so defined to resist inappropriate conceptions of our reality". Secondly, even if definitions can be agreed, since the prevalence and severity of ill-health varies in a complex and non-linear fashion with age, it is difficult to find comparable health surveys with a large enough sample size to allow disaggregation to single-year age bands.

An estimate of the prevalence of disability in the adult population of Great Britain was provided in the national survey carried out in 1969 (Harris, 1971). In this survey, degree of disability was operationalised in terms of a series of questions concerning capacity for self-care. Responses were divided into four ranked categories ranging from very severely handicapped to impaired. In addition the General Household Survey (GHS) asked questions about adults with limiting long-standing illness, disability or infirmity between 1976 and 1989. The 1991 Census was the first Census to ask about long-term illness. Thus, for example, we calculated 5% of 33-year-old cohort members in the 1991 NCDS sweep to be disabled, compared with 6% of 30- to 44-year-olds reporting limiting long-standing illness in the 1991 Census and 10% of 16- to 44-year-olds reporting limiting long-standing illness in the 1991 GHS. Our breakdown into the categories of 'moderate ill-health' and 'some ill-health' compared less favourably with data from other sources because of the different definitions and time frames used. Here we calculated 13% of 33-year-old cohort members in the 1991 NCDS sweep to have moderate ill-health and a further 24% to have some ill-health, compared with a total of 23% of respondents in the 1991 GHS who reported non-limiting long-standing illness. (The 1991 Census did not ask about non-limiting long-standing illness.)

In 1984 a new OPCS survey of disability was commissioned by the (then) Department of Health and Social Security with the aim of providing accurate information about the number of disabled people in Britain and their different levels of severity. Four separate investigations were carried out in 1985 and 1988, covering adults and children in private households and in communal establishments. The survey established 10 disability categories for adults and children and the results were published in a total of six reports (Martin et al, 1988; Martin and White, 1988; Bone and Meltzer, 1989; Martin et al, 1989; Smyth and Robus, 1989; Meltzer et al, 1989). We know from these disability surveys that if disability is categorised into 10 categories of increasing severity then there are likely to be equal numbers of children (under 16) in each severity category, that is, there are equal numbers of

children with mild and very severe disabilities. By comparison the distribution of severity of disability and extreme ill-health in the adult population has a very different pattern; there are lots of adults with mild disabilities but very few with severe disabilities.

One partial comparison we can make is to compare the NCDS with the prevalence estimates of disability and limiting long-term illness from the 1991 Census Sample of Anonymised Records (SARs). However, definitional differences between these two surveys mean that they yield different results. Four per cent of the NCDS cohort were experiencing disability or limiting long-term illness at age 7. By age 11 this had increased to 12% of the cohort, whereas by age 16 the proportion of the cohort experiencing disability or limiting long-term illness had decreased again to 8%. For comparison, from SARs it appears that 3% of children at each of these ages were experiencing disability or limiting long-term illness in 1991.

In attempting this sort of comparison it is important to recognise a further complication. The age of a survey may also affect the prevalence rate of childhood ill-health. Thus, not only is the incidence of infectious disease among contemporary cohorts of children different from that for the NCDS cohort, the incidence of particular types of disability or ill-health may also have changed between the NCDS and later studies. In particular, there is some evidence that the prevalence of childhood disability may have gradually increased over the past 30 years. Figure 1 shows the change in the rates of limiting long-standing illness in children (after smoothing) as recorded in the GHS between 1974 and 1995.

A final point worth noting when seeking to compare the NCDS measures with those from elsewhere is the importance of geography. Sutherland and Chesson (1994) highlight the need for local as well as national statistics. They found, for example, that the percentage of disabled people with respiratory disorders ranged from 13% in the OPCS disability surveys to 25% in a local study in the Grampian area. The fact that the NCDS takes a complete cohort as its sample may produce estimates of the prevalence of ill-health and disability which depart from those of other surveys which are designed to be nationally representative on the basis of some criteria other than birth rate or the local population of children.

Figure 1: Changes in limiting long-standing illness rates for children between 1974 and 1995 (smoothed* GHS data)

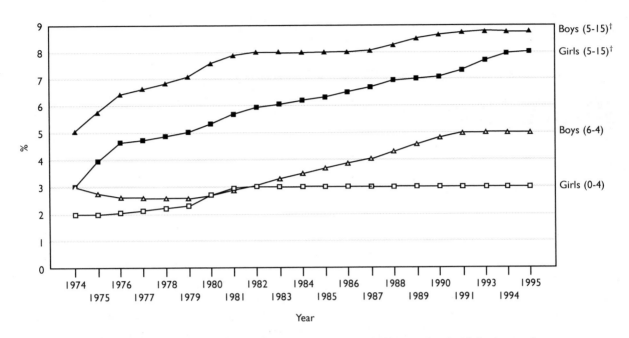

Notes: * The rates have been treated with a standard resistant smoother (4253H, twice) to highlight the trends.
† Between 1974 and 1978 this age group was 5-14.

Source: General Household Survey (1974-95)

4

Linking overcrowding with infectious and respiratory disease

The overall objective of this research topic is to examine the impact of overcrowding on respiratory health and infectious disease. While the key questions to be addressed by the study have been outlined in Chapter 1, a specific aim is to achieve a greater understanding of the impact of both childhood and present circumstances of overcrowding, as well as people's experiences and exposures to risk in the intervening period.

In attempting to overcome the possible deficiencies of previous studies, this study adopts two novel approaches to understanding the impact of overcrowding on respiratory health and infectious disease. Firstly, following the notion of the life-course, we are concerned to trace the pathways that the subjects of the NCDS took through the six data point to the age of 33. The objective here is to assess whether the impact of overcrowding upon health can be interpreted in an 'accumulation of risk' framework. Secondly, chi-squared automatic interaction detector (CHAID) analysis, a classification tree technique (see Appendix B), has been conducted to show the relative significance of overcrowding at different stages of the life-course. It helps illustrate whether current overcrowding is more important in affecting health than overcrowding at earlier points in the cohort member's life-course.

The extent of overcrowding

The first part of the analysis was to establish the extent of overcrowding (defined as more than one person per room) among NCDS cohort members in both childhood and adulthood. Figure 2 shows that the proportion of the cohort members of the NCDS experiencing overcrowding in childhood was high. In 1958, 32% of cohort members were living in overcrowded circumstances. While rates of overcrowding increased in years 7 (42%) and 11 (39%), by the age of 16 overcrowding was at 35%. Overcrowding fell dramatically at the age of 23 to 3%, before rising again to 12% at age 33.

This pattern of overcrowding among NCDS subjects is compared with evidence from SARs in Figure 2. The absolute levels of overcrowding in 1991 were much lower, but they display a similar pattern across most of the relevant age range. The most noticeable divergence is at the lower ages where SARs exhibit relatively stable levels of overcrowding from birth to age 7 while the NCDS indicates that the proportion of cohort members in overcrowded accommodation increased quite sharply. The explanation for this difference may well lie in a cohort effect in relation to the postwar baby boom and the changing household: dwelling balance over the postwar period. The decline in crowding in later childhood is much more gradual among the subjects of the NCDS than the SARs, but from ages 16 to 23 overcrowding in the NCDS drops very sharply to below the level recorded by SARs for those aged 23.

The experience of overcrowding over time

The pathways of crowding experienced by the NCDS cohort members are presented in Figures 3(a) and 3(b). Because each cohort member is classified using a variable which draws on

Figure 2: Overcrowding by age

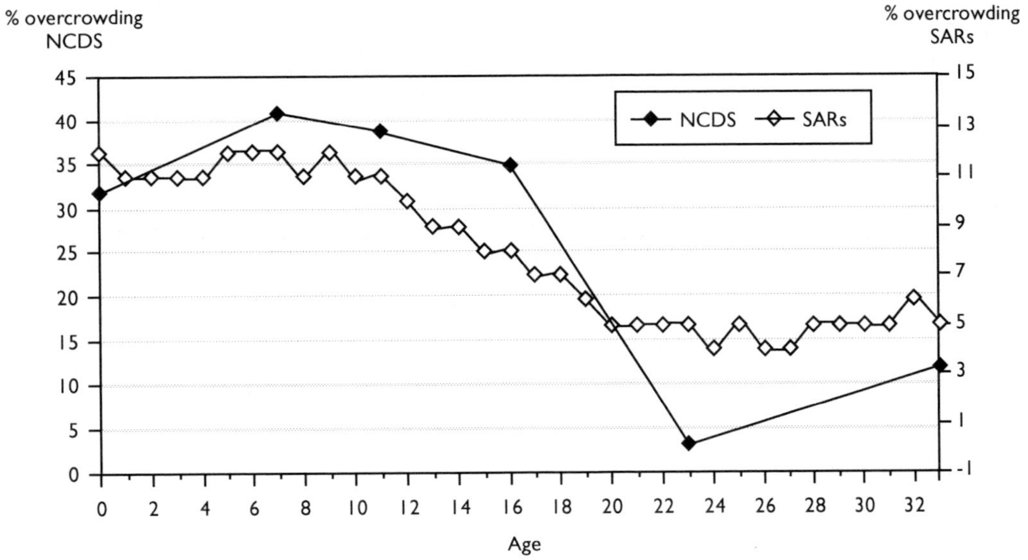

Source: NCDS; 1991 Census Sample of Anonymised Records

experience of crowding at each sweep, the data demands of this analysis are high. This is witnessed by the fact that by sweep 5 the initial sample of 16,920 had been reduced to 5,194.

By far the most frequent pathway through to age 33 involves no overcrowding. Over one third (40%) of the subjects had not been crowded at any point to age 33. At the other end of the spectrum, although 14% of subjects were crowded throughout childhood the number of subjects crowded at all data points was negligible. Indeed, age 23 represents a clear transition – as one might expect in terms of new household formation – when the overall rate of overcrowding decreases to only 3%, compared to 35% at age 16. Thus, most of those who were overcrowded at 16 moved to a non-crowded state by the age of 23.

Between the two extremes a diverse range of pathways were followed. At the most general level there tended to be a fair degree of continuity between sweeps, in as much as crowding status at one sweep is quite a good indicator of crowding status in the next sweep. The pathways also suggest that cohort members who moved from an overcrowded to a non-overcrowded state showed a relatively low propensity to return to crowding.

Overcrowding and ill-health

Bivariate analysis involving the calculation of odds ratios was conducted to assess the link between overcrowding and respiratory health and infectious disease. The odds of those in each overcrowding pathway experiencing respiratory health problems and infectious disease were calculated for each sweep relative to the reference group of cohort members who had not experienced overcrowding.

Overall, very few of the calculated odds ratios formally achieve statistical significance at the 5% level so in many cases it is not possible to reject the hypothesis that living in overcrowded conditions has no effect upon these measures of ill-health. None the less, the pathways exhibit results which warrant comment.

As indicated in Figures 3(a) and 3(b), when the analysis reaches sweeps 4 and 5 the number of subjects following some of the pathways is very small. In these circumstances the low counts in the relevant cells of the tables upon which the odds ratios are based make the meaningful interpretation of odds ratios difficult. The odds ratios based upon very low counts have been marked in the figures.

Figure 3(a): Overcrowding pathway: overcrowded at birth

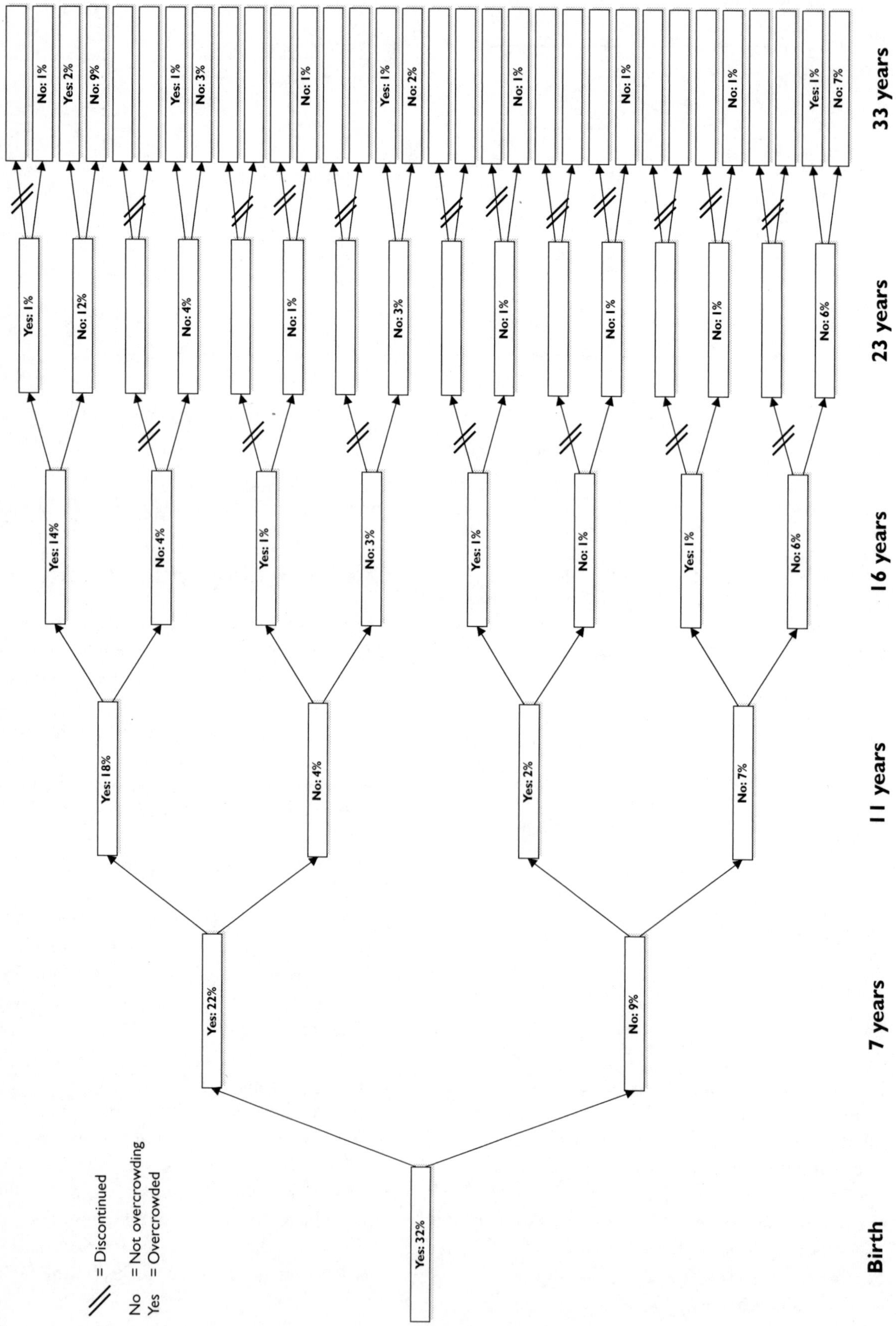

Legend:

/ / = Discontinued

No = Not overcrowding
Yes = Overcrowded

Columns (left to right): Birth | 7 years | 11 years | 16 years | 23 years | 33 years

Birth: Yes: 32%

7 years: Yes: 22%; No: 9%

11 years: Yes: 18%; No: 4%; Yes: 2%; No: 7%

16 years: Yes: 14%; No: 4%; Yes: 1%; No: 3%; Yes: 1%; No: 1%; Yes: 1%; No: 6%

23 years: Yes: 1%; No: 12%; No: 4%; No: 1%; No: 3%; No: 1%; No: 1%; No: 1%; No: 6%

33 years: No: 1%; Yes: 2%; No: 9%; Yes: 1%; No: 3%; No: 1%; Yes: 1%; No: 2%; No: 1%; No: 1%; No: 1%; Yes: 1%; No: 7%

Figure 3(b): Overcrowding pathway: not overcrowded at birth

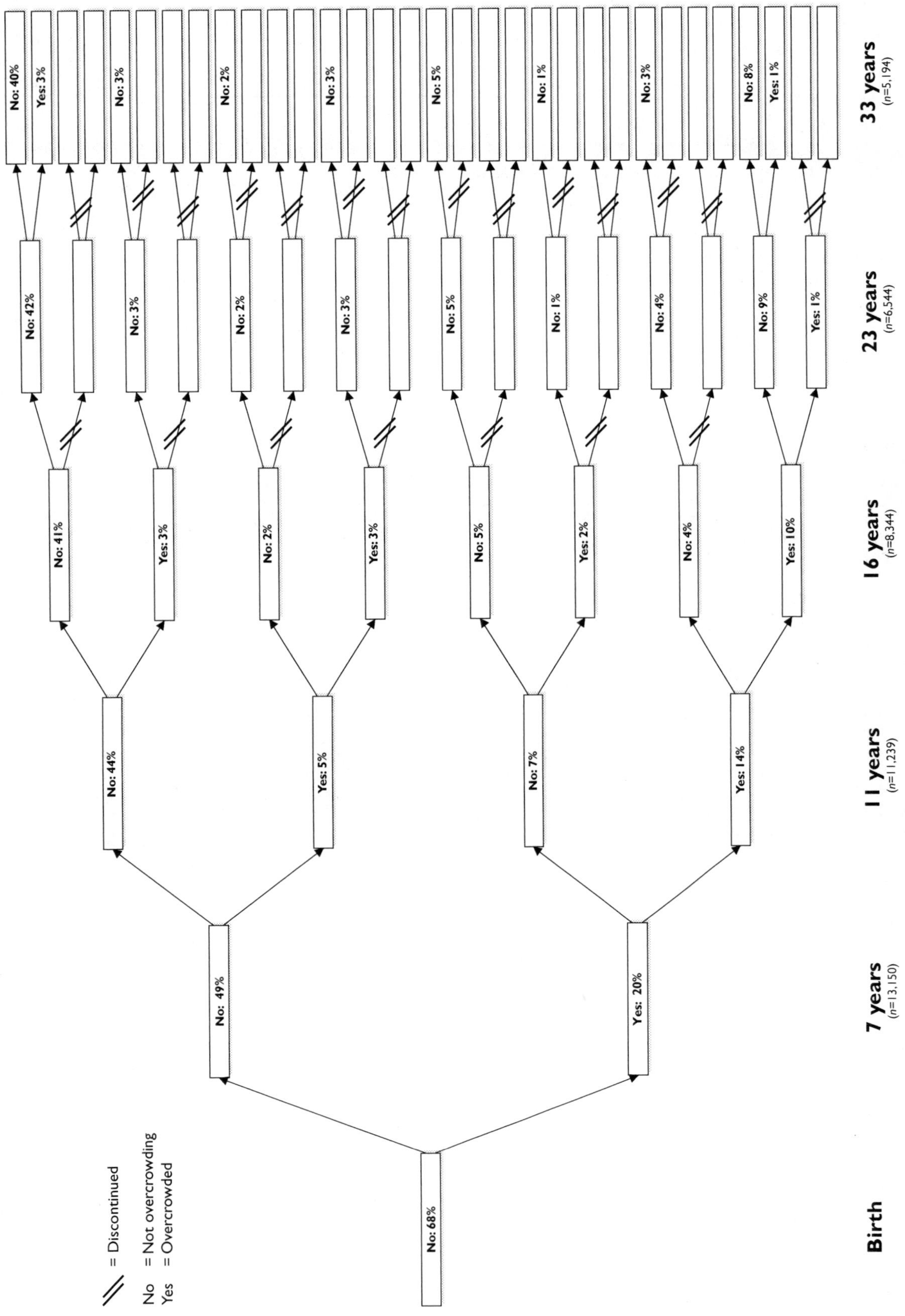

// = Discontinued

No = Not overcrowding
Yes = Overcrowded

| Birth | 7 years (n=13,150) | 11 years (n=11,239) | 16 years (n=8,344) | 23 years (n=6,544) | 33 years (n=5,194) |

Figure 4(a): Respiratory disease by overcrowding pathways (odds ratios): overcrowded at birth

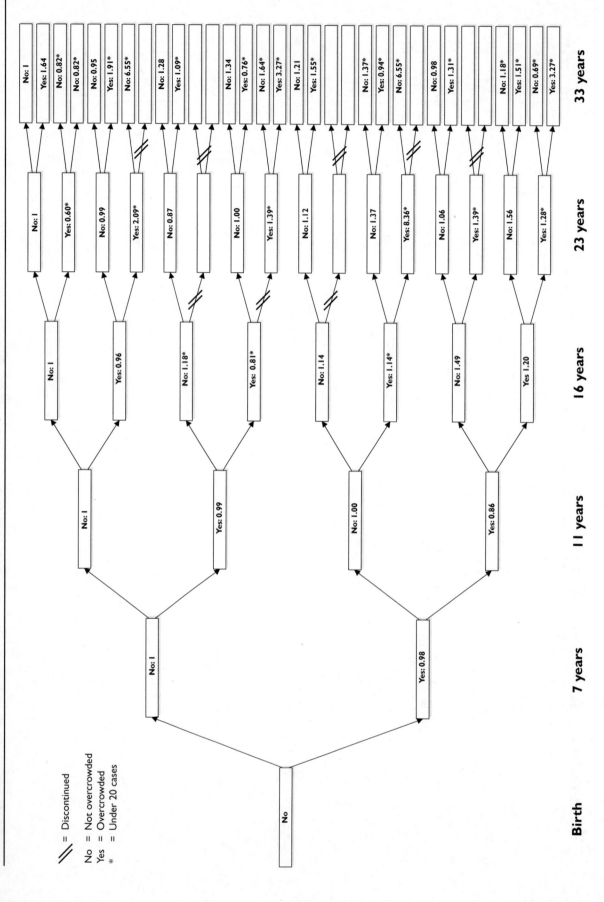

Figure 4(b): Respiratory disease by overcrowding pathway (odds ratios): not overcrowded at birth

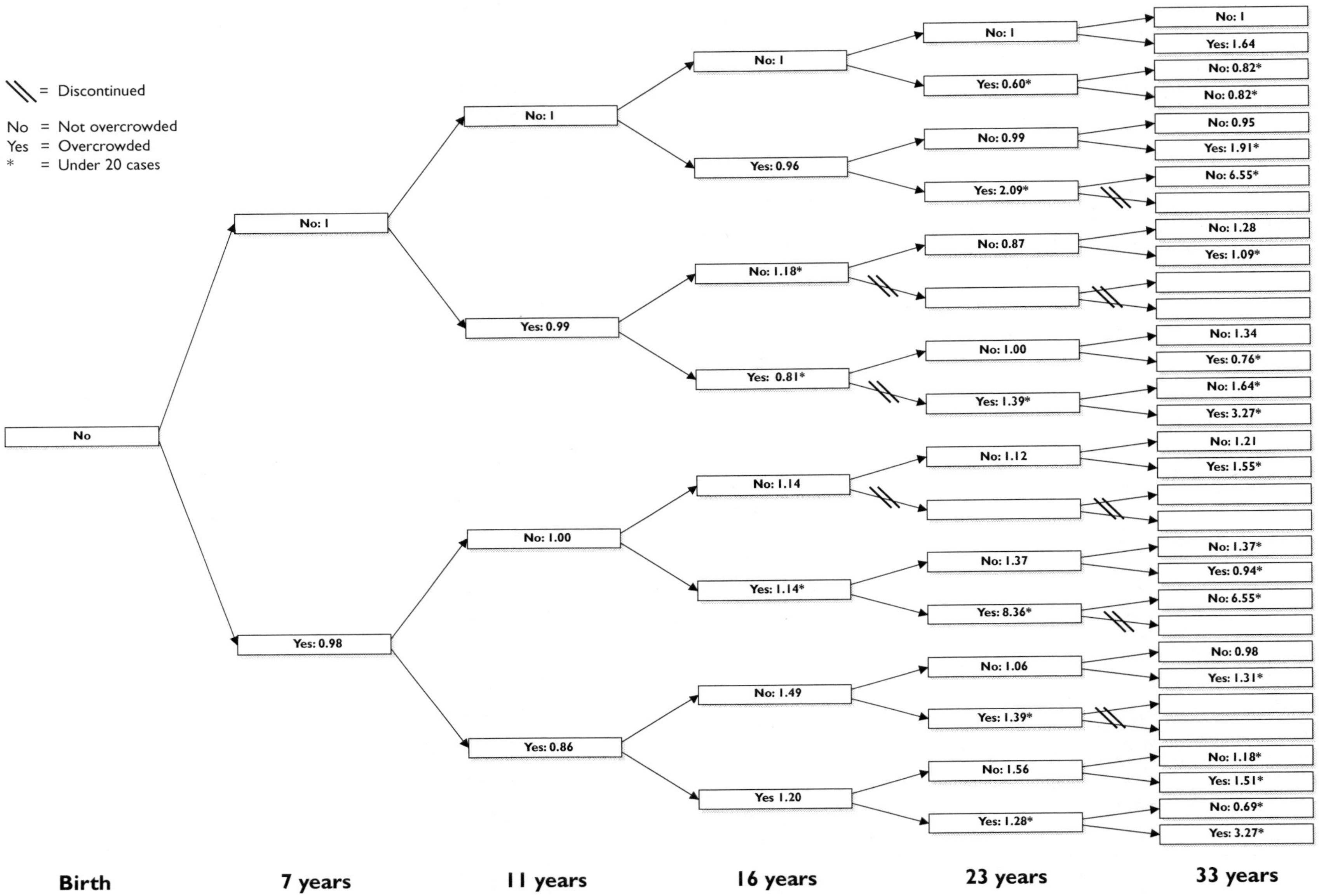

// = Discontinued

No = Not overcrowded
Yes = Overcrowded
* = Under 20 cases

Birth   7 years   11 years   16 years   23 years   33 years

Respiratory disease

Figures 4(a) and 4(b) reproduce the pathways diagram and present the odds of cohort members in a particular pathway experiencing respiratory disease.

At sweep 1 cohort members who had experienced overcrowding at birth but who may or not have also experienced overcrowding at 7 showed odds ratios greater than one relative to the reference category (those who had not been overcrowded either at birth or age 7). This suggests that those who had experienced overcrowding at birth were more likely to have experienced some form of respiratory illness by age 7, than those who had not experienced overcrowding at birth.

The picture in sweep 2 becomes more complex. While being overcrowded at birth, age 7 and 11 results in an odds ratio of less than one, the highest odds ratios are shown for those NCDS subjects who had experienced overcrowding at birth, but not at age 7 and who may or may not have experienced overcrowding at 11. On the other hand, all groups of cohort members who had not experienced overcrowding at birth, whatever their experience of crowding at 7 and 11, had odds ratios of one or less.

A similarly complex relationship between overcrowding and respiratory disease emerges in sweeps 3 to 5 and interpretation of the results is complicated by the fact that a number of the pathways are exhausted as you move through the sweeps. All but one of the odds ratios for pathways with more than 20 cases at sweep 3 are greater than one, with the highest ratio (1.49) recorded by those experiencing crowding at age 7 and 11, but not at birth and 16. This indicates that all cohort members who experienced overcrowding at some point had a greater likelihood of experiencing respiratory disease at 16 than those who were never overcrowded, with the exception of those whose first experience of overcrowding was at age 16.

Following the pathways through to sweep 4 indicates that those who were crowded across ages 7, 11 and 16 continued to exhibit relatively high odds ratios at age 23 – indeed those crowded at every age to 23 recorded the highest odds ratio (1.78) – while those who had been crowded at 7

and 11 but not 16 saw their experience polarise: the odds ratio for those who had also been crowded at birth remained high (1.50) while the odds ratio for those who had not been crowded at birth dropped back to 1.06.

These observations could be read as providing support for a version of the accumulated risk model linking housing and health. Cohort members crowded at birth, 7 and 11 had accumulated sufficient 'risk' that they still had a higher likelihood of respiratory disease at age 23, while those not crowded at birth could 'recover' from crowding at 7 and 11 by age 23. This interpretation is complicated by the observation that the second highest odds ratio at age 23 is in fact recorded by those who were crowded at birth and age 7 but not crowded subsequently (1.58) and that the pathway running from overcrowding at birth and no subsequent overcrowding shows a relatively high set of odds ratios throughout childhood, even if the ratio declines at 23. Indeed, an accumulation of risk interpretation of the pathways is rendered further problematic by the observation that those whose only experience of crowding is at birth exhibit greater likelihood of respiratory ill-health during childhood than those crowded at all of the first three sweeps. This observation could, in contrast, be interpreted as indicating that the period around birth is a particularly 'critical period' in a person's development during which adverse housing conditions are particularly damaging to later health.

Those pathways that still yield meaningful results in sweep 5 mostly relate to those who were not crowded at 33 and in most cases the odds ratio is greater than one. The exception is those who are crowded from birth to age 16, not crowded at 23, but return to crowded conditions at 33. This group recorded the substantial odds ratio of 2.18. Thus, relative to those who have never been crowded, most of these groups showed an increased likelihood of experiencing respiratory ill-health.

Overall, no clear pattern emerges from the pathways analysis regarding the likelihood of subjects who experience overcrowding in childhood suffering respiratory ill-health in childhood and/or later life. The analysis does not lend unambiguous support to one particular interpretation of the association between the two variables: there is limited evidence

Figure 5(a): Infectious diseases by overcrowding pathway (odds ratios): overcrowded at birth

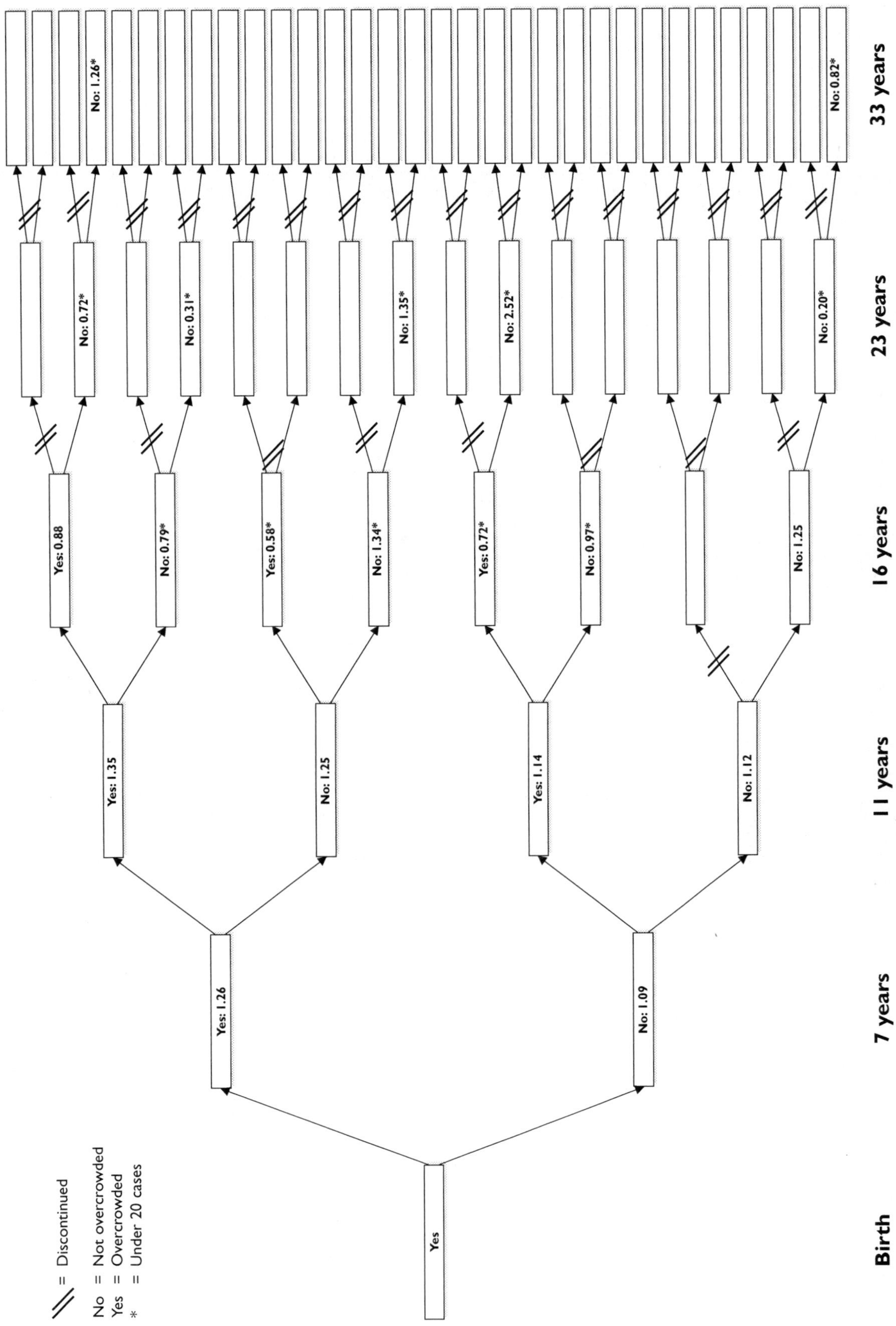

Figure 5(b): Infectious diseases by overcrowding pathway (odds ratios): not overcrowded at birth

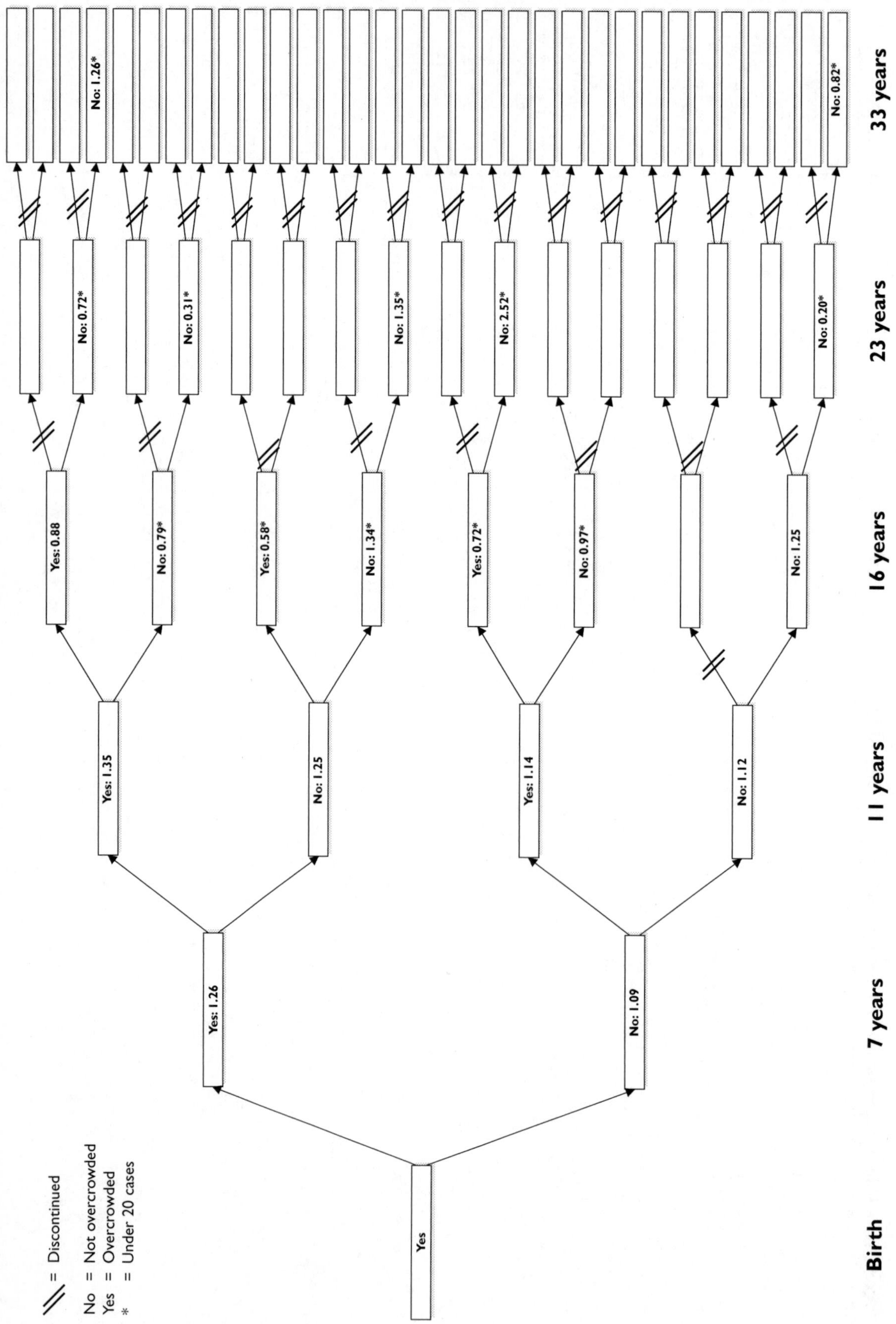

/ = Discontinued

No = Not overcrowded
Yes = Overcrowded
* = Under 20 cases

Birth | 7 years | 11 years | 16 years | 23 years | 33 years

Yes

Yes: 1.26

No: 1.09

Yes: 1.35

No: 1.25

Yes: 1.14

No: 1.12

Yes: 0.88

No: 0.79*

Yes: 0.58*

No: 1.34*

Yes: 0.72*

No: 0.97*

No: 1.25

No: 0.72*

No: 0.31*

No: 1.35*

No: 2.52*

No: 0.20*

No: 1.26*

No: 0.82*

to support the accumulation of risk interpretation of the link between crowding and respiratory ill-health, but from this relatively simple analysis other interpretations of the link appear equally plausible.

Infectious disease

The experience of infectious disease of those on different overcrowding pathways is presented in Figures 5(a) and 5(b). In reading these figures it is important to recall that for ages 7 and 11 the measure relates to experience of infectious disease at any time prior to the data collection point, while for ages 16, 23, and 33 to particular experiences of infectious disease in the last year (for details see Chapter 3). The common childhood infectious diseases, which for the cohort members were almost universally experienced, were excluded from the analysis.

The figures show that the odds ratios are more than one for all categories at sweep 1, although the risks of experiencing infectious disease was highest for those subjects who were overcrowded at both birth and age 7 (1.26). At sweep 2, odds ratios greater than one can be seen for all categories of subjects born in overcrowded circumstances regardless of whether they were overcrowded at later stages in childhood. Again the highest odds ratios were experienced by those who were overcrowded throughout their childhood (1.35), while the lowest risks were experienced by those who were currently overcrowded (that is, at age 11) but had not suffered from overcrowding conditions at either birth or 7 (0.97).

No clear picture emerges from the results at sweeps 3 through to 5 and the very small proportion of the NCDS cohort members experiencing infectious disease after the age of 11 means that the counts in each pathway are too small to give meaningful results. Recognising that any interpretation must be treated with considerable caution, therefore, it appears that the strong pattern that previously existed between overcrowded conditions and risk of infection no longer holds. Many of the odds ratios are substantially lower than one, which would suggest that those suffering overcrowding at some point in time are less likely to experience infectious disease than those who have never been overcrowded. It is interesting to note, however, that

one of the strongest pathways through the data is again crowded at birth and no subsequent crowding and that cohort members following this route recorded an odds ratio greater than one at 16 (1.25) while those overcrowded throughout childhood recorded an odds ratio below one. Conversely those who were not crowded at birth but had been crowded at every sweep since then recorded odds ratios greater than one at all sweeps.

Again these observations lend limited support to a model of the link between disease and housing which focuses on an accumulation of risk. They could be read as indicating that infectious disease in childhood is linked to current and/or recent overcrowding, but that by the age of 16 experience of infectious disease is only loosely related to this dimension of housing circumstances.

Chi-squared automatic interaction detector analysis

This section details the results of the impact of overcrowding on respiratory ill-health at the ages of 23 and 33 using CHAID analysis. It was not possible to conduct a CHAID analysis in relation to infectious disease because of the small proportion of subjects experiencing infectious disease in adulthood.

Chi-squared automatic interaction detector analysis predicts which groups of people experience the highest risk of respiratory health problems. It allows both the combination of categories within variables and the sorting of variables to produce statistically significant results. The technique allows for the identification of sub-groups with particularly high risks of respiratory disease (as well as low rates).

Figure 6 shows the most statistically significant overcrowding variables affecting the risk of respiratory disease at the age of 23. The boxes show the sample size of the sub-group and the percentage of that sub-group that suffer a respiratory disease. Twenty-one per cent of NCDS subjects ($n=5,194$) were suffering from a respiratory disease at 23. Overcrowding at the age of 7 was the most statistically significant factor affecting this group's risk. Thus, one in four of those overcrowded at the age of 7 suffered from a respiratory disease at the

Figure 6: Experience of respiratory disease at the age of 23 by overcrowding

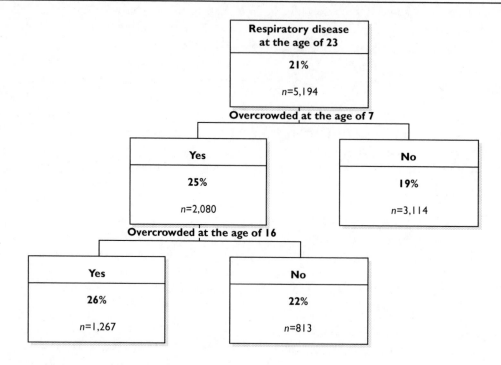

Figure 7: Experience of respiratory disease at the age of 33 by overcrowding

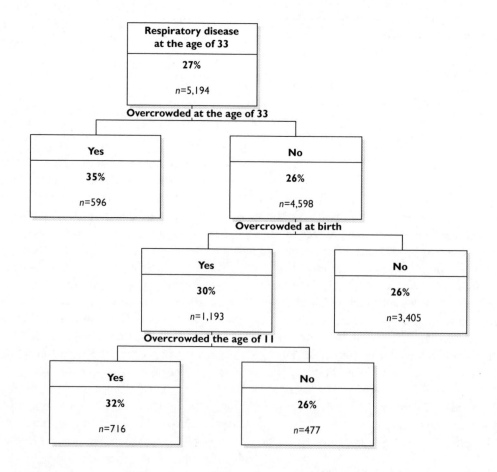

age of 23 (25%). This group can be further sub-divided by whether they were also overcrowded at the age of 16. Risks of respiratory disease increased slightly for those who, in addition to being overcrowded at the age of 7, were also overcrowded at the age of 16 (26%).

Current circumstances are more statistically significant in predicting a cohort member's risk of respiratory disease at the age of 33. Figure 7 shows that while 27% of NCDS cohort members experienced respiratory disease at the age of 33, those who were living in overcrowded conditions at this age had much higher risks of respiratory disease (35%). The figure also demonstrates people not overcrowded at 33, but who had nevertheless experienced overcrowding some time in their lives, had higher risks of respiratory disease. Thus, subjects who were not overcrowded at 33, but who had been overcrowded at birth and at 11 had a risk of respiratory disease of 32%. This observation may lend support to some form of 'critical period' interpretation of the link between health and housing. Such an interpretation would argue that there are particular stages in a person's development during which it is particularly harmful to later health to experience adverse housing conditions.

Summary

This chapter has briefly examined the impact of overcrowding over the life-course on respiratory health and infectious disease. It has traced the different pathways of overcrowding and explored the likelihood of experiencing poor respiratory health and infectious disease associated with each pathway.

The cohort members followed a complex set of housing pathways with 60% experiencing overcrowding at least once between birth and age 33. Overall the picture which emerges from the pathway analysis with respect to health is not open to simple interpretation.

Current overcrowding is not always associated with a raised probability of respiratory ill-health, although the CHAID analysis highlights current overcrowding as being important in relation to the respiratory health of the cohort members at 33.

Overcrowding in a number of consecutive sweeps appears to raise the likelihood of respiratory ill-health in later childhood and adulthood. This may be seen as supporting an accumulation of risk interpretation of the link between housing deprivation and health. Yet the fact that those who were overcrowded at birth but not in later sweeps exhibited some of the highest probabilities of ill-health suggests that if an accumulation of risks framework is a sensible approach then it is likely that the range of risks incorporated into the analysis needs to be extended. It should include other aspects of housing, such as damp or mould, which have been linked with respiratory disease and which are not necessarily closely related to overcrowding, and it should go beyond housing to examine other aspects of life-style and circumstances.

That current overcrowding comes to play a more dominant role than crowding in earlier life once the cohort members reach 33 also appears to count against a straightforward accumulation of housing risk model. An equally interesting aspect of the analysis of respiratory ill-health at age 33 is that, for those who are not overcrowded at 33, an experience of overcrowding at birth and age 11 increased the likelihood of suffering from illness at 33. This suggests that housing history matters: even though they may be adequately housed in adulthood those who had experienced adverse housing conditions in earlier life were still more likely to be ill than had they been adequately accommodated throughout.

It appears that cohort members who experience overcrowding in early childhood are generally more likely to experience infectious disease than those who have never been overcrowded. But that picture becomes less clear for later sweeps. There is no strong indication that crowding continues to be a key to understanding the increased likelihood of infectious disease once the cohort members reach age 16. There is also little sign that crowding in early life has the effect of increasing the odds of experiencing infectious disease in later childhood or early adulthood.

5

The impact of timing and duration of housing deprivation on health

In this chapter we consider the derivation of a housing deprivation index from the NCDS data. We then examine whether NCDS cohort members who followed different housing deprivation pathways to age 33 displayed different likelihoods of experiencing severe or moderate ill-health.

Housing deprivation and morbidity: deriving the housing deprivation index

A key element of this study was to explore the scope for devising a reliable and valid housing deprivation index that can be used to study the effects that 'bad' housing conditions have on health. But what is the best way to construct a housing deprivation index? This question can be divided into two parts. Firstly, what, if anything, does the index measure? Secondly, which of the many potential indices provides the most accurate and precise measurement? Answering these questions is far from simple. It is also a task which is not attempted as often as it might be in the existing literature. Several studies have made use of housing deprivation indices and/or combinations of indicators of housing deprivation when examining the distribution of mortality and morbidity in the population. However, the indicators that have been used and the way that housing deprivation indices have been constructed have varied from one study to the next (see Murie, 1983; Lee et al, 1995 for discussion), and theoretical discussions on the nature and measurement of deprivation are often dealt with in a cursory manner or are entirely absent. Indeed, many deprivation indices seem to be composed of combinations of variables that the authors think measure something 'bad', although what this 'bad' thing is is often unclear. Various statistical procedures and transformations are often performed on the components of the index, usually in order to ensure equal weighting, that is, so that each variable provides an equal contribution to the final index. Yet, the justification for such statistical procedures is frequently absent. The terms 'deprivation' and 'multiple deprivation' are generally used loosely, with little reference to the specific technical meanings of these terms.

The theory of poverty and deprivation

In order to measure housing deprivation and/or poverty more accurately, it is necessary to be precise about the meaning of these terms. First, one needs to distinguish between 'absolute' and 'relative' poverty. The 'absolute' concept of poverty is dominated by the individual's requirements for physiological efficiency. It is a very limited conception of human needs, especially when considering that people are not just physical beings but social beings who play a number of roles in society. They have obligations as workers, parents, neighbours, friends and citizens that they are expected to meet and which they themselves want to meet. Studies of people's behaviour after they have experienced a drastic cut in resources show that they sometimes act to fulfil their social obligations before they act to satisfy their physical wants. They require income to fulfil their various roles and participate in the social customs and associations to which they have become habituated and not only to satisfy their physical wants (Townsend and Gordon, 1993).

Deprivation and poverty, like evolution, are both scientific and moral concepts. Many of the problems of measuring arise because the moral and scientific concepts are often confused. In scientific terms, a person or household in Britain is 'poor' when they have both a low standard of living and a low income. They are not poor if they have a low income and a reasonable standard of living or if they have a low standard of living but a high income. Both low income and low standard of living can only be accurately measured relative to the norms of the person's or household's society.

A low standard of living is often measured by using a deprivation index (high deprivation equals a low standard of living) or by consumption expenditure (low consumption expenditure equals a low standard of living). Of these two methods, deprivation indices are more accurate since consumption expenditure is often only measured over a brief period and is obviously not independent of available income (Gordon and Pantazis, 1997).

This 'scientific' concept of poverty can be made universally applicable by using the broader concept of resources instead of just monetary income. Poverty can then be defined as the point at which resources are so seriously below those commanded by the average individual or family that the poor are, in effect, excluded from ordinary living patterns, customs and activities. As resources for any individual or family are diminished, there is a point at which there occurs a sudden withdrawal from participation in the customs and activities sanctioned by the culture. The point at which withdrawal escalates disproportionately to falling resources can be defined as the poverty line or threshold (Townsend, 1979, 1993).

There is no official government definition of poverty in Britain; however, the British government was a signatory to the following European Commission definition of poverty which was adopted on the 19 December 1984 (EEC, 1985, 1991):

The poor shall be taken to mean persons, families and groups of persons whose resources (material, cultural and social) are so limited as to exclude them from the minimum acceptable way of life in the Member State in which they live.

This 'relative' concept of poverty is now widely accepted (Piachaud, 1987); however; it is not easy to measure poverty directly (Atkinson, 1985a, 1985b; Lewis and Ulph, 1988) but it is possible to obtain measures of 'deprivation'. These two concepts are tightly linked and there is general agreement that the concept of deprivation covers the various conditions, independent of income, experienced by people who are poor, while the concept of poverty refers to the lack of income and other resources which makes those conditions inescapable or at least highly likely (Townsend, 1987).

The measurement of poverty and deprivation

From these definitions, it is clear that in order to measure poverty/deprivation accurately, surveys or censuses must be used that establish both the 'normal' or 'average' standard of living of the majority in a society/culture and any 'enforced' reductions in this standard due to lack of resources.

Social scientists have been using deprivation surveys to study poverty in Britain for over a hundred years. All these surveys have shown that certain groups are more likely to suffer from multiple housing deprivation than others (that is, lone parents and the unemployed are not equally likely to be living in poverty and indices that consider them to be are probably wrong). Survey-based deprivation indices that give equal weight to their component variables are therefore likely to yield inaccurate results.

Since many survey-based deprivation indices are generally composed of both direct and surrogate or proxy measures of housing deprivation, there are two basic requirements they should fulfil to ensure accuracy (Gordon, 1995):

- The components of the index should be weighted to reflect the different probability that each group has of suffering from multiple housing deprivation; and
- The components of the index must be additive, for example, if an index is composed of two variables, overcrowding and damp, then researchers must be confident that children living

in damp overcrowded households are likely to be 'more deprived' than either children in overcrowded households without damp or children in damp households which are not overcrowded.

In order to construct an aggregate housing deprivation index it is necessary to demonstrate that each of its components are both reliable and valid measures of housing deprivation. Each component in the index needs to be a valid predictor of 'poor' health both in isolation and combination.

In order to examine the validity of the various components of a housing deprivation index, binary, ordinal and nominal logistic regression were employed. These techniques are designed for the analysis of categorical data such as the health index. Each technique differs slightly in its assumptions about the distribution of the data, but each examines the association between a dependent health variable and, in the current instance, indicators of housing circumstances. The techniques seek to estimate the probability of cohort members in different health categories being in different housing circumstances and then test whether any differences in these likelihoods are statistically significant. Further details of the methods used and the rationale for using them are provided in Appendix B.

Housing deprivation in the NCDS

In this section we examine the components of a housing deprivation index for each of the sweeps of the NCDS separately and consider the extent to which the NCDS cohort members have experienced housing deprivation in each sweep. The analysis starts with the 1965 sweep of the NCDS because the only housing-related information collected in the 1958 sweep was overcrowding and therefore it is not possible to construct an index of housing deprivation for that sweep.

Housing deprivation in 1965

Four different types of logistic regression model were estimated for each variable in the 1965 sweep of the NCDS that could potentially be used as part of a housing deprivation index. The variables are:

- housing difficulties recorded by the health visitor;
- not having sole access to hot water;
- overcrowding (more than one person per room);
- lacking or having to share an indoor toilet;
- not having sole access to a bath;
- living in non self-contained accommodation (rooms, caravans, etc);
- not having sole access to a garden or yard;
- not having sole access to a cooker;
- living in a flat.

All of these are 'objective' characteristics of the cohort member's housing circumstances with the exception of the first, which is clearly the health visitor's subjective assessment of difficulties. Such assessments were not conducted blind and therefore it is conceivable that whether the cohort member was deemed to have been in housing difficulty may have been influenced by whether they had a disability or severe health problem. However, there is no indication that their assessment was affected by the cohort member's health condition, nor is there any reason to doubt the health visitor's professionalism. Indeed, they appear to have erred on the side of caution with regard to measuring housing deprivation. Summary tables for the analysis are presented in Appendix C.

The housing deprivation variable that was the most significant predictor of 'poor' health in the 1965 sweep of the NCDS was the health visitor's assessment that the cohort member's family was suffering from housing difficulties (Appendix C, Table 1). There was (on average) a 46% greater chance (odds of 1.46 to 1) that if the health visitor recorded that there were housing difficulties the cohort member would also suffer from disability or severe or moderate ill-health.

The analysis demonstrates that the health visitor's assessment of housing difficulties is not a significant predictor of the difference between 'no health problems' and 'minor health problems'. However, it is a highly significant predictor of 'no health problems' versus 'moderate health problems' and 'no health problems' versus 'disability/severe health problems'. There is (on average) a 74% greater chance that a cohort member experienced disability or severe health problems in 1965 if the health visitor recorded housing difficulties compared with the chance that they experienced 'no health problems' (Appendix C, Table 1).

All nine housing variables recorded on the 1965 NCDS are positively associated with an increased chance (odds) of 'poor' health with the exception of 'living in a flat' (Appendix C, Table 9). However, the results for living in non-self-contained accommodation (rooms, caravans, etc) (Appendix C, Table 6), not having sole access to a garden or yard (Appendix C, Table 7) and not having sole access to a cooker (Appendix C, Table 8) were not statistically significant at the 5% level.

Reliability analysis for housing deprivation variables at age seven

All measurement is subject to error that can take the form of either random variations or systematic bias (Stanley, 1971, lists many causes of bias). Random errors of measurement can never be completely eliminated. However, if the error is only small relative to the size of the phenomena being studied, then the measurement will be reliable. Reliable measurements are repeatable; they have a high degree of precision.

One way of examining the reliability of an index is to use Cronbach's coefficient alpha, which assesses the average correlation between sets of questions and ranges from 0 (indicating poor reliability) to 1 (indicating 100% reliability). (See Appendix B for more detail.)

Coefficient alpha is 0.688 for the nine questions in the 1965 sweep of the NCDS. Nunnally (1981) argues that in the early stages of research, reliability of 0.70 or higher is sufficient. Therefore, the nine NCDS 1965 sweep housing deprivation questions have a reasonably high degree of reliability. However, it would be desirable to increase the reliability if possible without compromising the validity of the housing deprivation scale.

Coefficient alpha can also be used to test the reliability of individual questions. Table 8 shows how the alpha coefficient would change if any single question were deleted from the housing deprivation index.

Table 8: Reliability of the nine housing deprivation questions: 1965 sweep

Variable	Scale mean if item deleted	Scale variance if item deleted	Corrected item – total correlation	Alpha if item deleted
HVISIT65	0.9948	1.7547	0.4491	0.6478
HOTW65	0.9846	1.6529	0.5681	0.6233
CROWD65	**0.6526**	**1.5976**	**0.2296**	**0.7255**
LAV65	0.9020	1.5356	0.4945	0.6301
BATH65	0.9473	1.5195	0.6305	0.6001
NOTSELF65	1.0311	1.9614	0.2565	0.6810
YARD65	0.9716	1.6965	0.4526	0.6439
COOK65	1.0575	2.0489	0.2683	0.6867
FLATS65	**0.9835**	**1.9399**	**0.1446**	**0.7007**

Number of cases = 13,535   Number of items = 9
Cronbach's alpha for the nine questions = 0.6879

Removing either of the two questions highlighted in bold would increase coefficient alpha above 0.70. Deleting the overcrowding question would result in the greatest increase in alpha. However, this would decrease the validity of the housing deprivation index since the logistic regression models have demonstrated that overcrowding is strongly associated with ill-health (see Appendix C, Table 3). Yet while overcrowding is a valid measure of housing deprivation in the 1965 sweep it is an unreliable measure because cohort members living in overcrowded accommodation were unlikely to be experiencing other types of housing deprivation. Overcrowding is 'unreliable' because it measures a different aspect of housing deprivation from the other variables. When deciding which variables to include in any index a trade-off often has to be made between increased reliability or validity: a 'good' index is one that manages to achieve a balance between the two.

In contrast to overcrowding, removing the measure of children living in flats would increase both alpha to above 0.70 and also the validity of the scale, since living in flats was not positively associated with an increased risk of 'poor' health (see Appendix C, Table 9). The final housing deprivation index for sweep 1 of the NCDS should thus consist of eight variables and a Cronbach's alpha of 0.7007.

Housing deprivation in 1969

Logistic regression models were estimated for each of the 16 variables in the 1969 sweep of the NCDS that could potentially be used as part of a housing deprivation index. The variables are:

- Mother of cohort member unsatisfied or very unsatisfied with the accommodation.
- Mother of cohort member unsatisfied with location of accommodation.
- Living in a flat.
- Front door of the accommodation on or above the third floor of the building.
- Mother of cohort member unsatisfied with comfort, manageability or 'ease of running' of the accommodation.
- Mother of cohort member unsatisfied with other aspects of accommodation.
- Living in non-self-contained accommodation (rooms, caravans, etc).
- Cohort member has to share a bed with others.
- Mother of cohort member unsatisfied with size of accommodation.
- Not having sole access to hot water.
- Mother of cohort member unsatisfied with garden or outdoor play facilities.
- Overcrowding (more than one person per room).
- Not having sole access to a bath.
- Mother of cohort member unsatisfied with ownership (for example, 'our home') of accommodation.
- Lacking or having to share an indoor toilet.
- Not having sole access to a cooker.

There are twice as many potential housing deprivation questions in the 1969 sweep of the NCDS than there were in the 1965 sweep. This is mainly because a series of seven questions were asked of the cohort member's mother about her satisfaction with the accommodation. Summary tables for the analysis are presented in Appendix C, Tables 10-25.

As was the case with the 1965 sweep, the most powerful housing deprivation variables that were associated with 'poor' health in the 1969 sweep were those collecting subjective data. In this instance they were seeking information on perceptions of satisfaction with the accommodation. These questions were generally more 'powerful' than those that asked about lack of amenities or the physical nature of the accommodation. These results support Murie's (1983) suggestion that there is more to housing deprivation than just the lack of amenities or overcrowding.

All 16 variables are positively associated with an increased risk of 'poor' health. However, the variable 'Mother of cohort member unsatisfied with ownership (for example, "our home") of accommodation' (Appendix C, Table 23) 'Lacking or having to share an indoor toilet' (Appendix C, Table 24) and 'Not having sole access to a cooker' (Appendix C, Table 25) were not statistically significant at the 5% level. Thus, by the end of the 1960s these kind of questions addressing the absence of basic amenities (access to indoor toilets and adequate cooking facilities) were becoming relatively insensitive indicators of housing deprivation. Such questions had been used since the pioneering work of Charles Booth at the end of the 19th century to measure housing deprivation, but the slum-clearance and council house building programmes of the 1960s and 1970s had provided most of the population with at least these basic housing amenities.

Reliability analysis for housing deprivation variables at age 11

Table 9 shows the summary reliability results for the 16 potential housing deprivation questions in the 1969 sweep of the NCDS. The overall Cronbach's coefficient alpha for the 16 questions is 0.6163, which is less than the 0.70 level which is desirable. The main reason why the housing deprivation questions in the 1969 sweep of the NCDS are less reliable than those in the 1965 sweep is because the 16 1969 questions are measuring two slightly different aspects of housing deprivation. In addition to the usual 'lack of basic amenities'-type questions there is the set of questions relating to the cohort member's mother's perceptions of the family's housing conditions. It seems highly probable that the cohort member's mothers are concerned about considerably more than just 'basic amenities' and 'overcrowding' when assessing the quality and suitability of their accommodation.

Table 9: Reliability of the 16 housing deprivation questions: 1969 sweep

Variable	Scale mean if item deleted	Scale variance if item deleted	Corrected item – total correlation	Alpha if item deleted
BATH69	1.3231	2.2894	0.4480	0.5697
BED69	1.2167	2.2737	0.2350	0.6046
COMFOR69	1.3005	2.3700	0.2683	0.5954
COOK69	1.3813	2.6323	0.1744	0.6130
CROWD11	0.9960	2.0005	0.3209	0.5926
FLATS69	1.3007	2.4573	0.1650	0.6122
GARDEN69	1.3668	2.6143	0.1035	0.6156
HIRISE69	1.3701	2.6085	0.1346	0.6133
HOTW69	1.3466	2.3948	0.4056	0.5824
LAV69	1.2802	2.2423	0.3712	0.5761
LOCATION69	**1.3391**	**2.5617**	**0.1083**	**0.6171**
NOTSELF69	1.3727	2.5879	0.2061	0.6086
OTHER69	**1.3238**	**2.5418**	**0.1036**	**0.6192**
OWNER69	**1.3738**	**2.6653**	**0.0084**	**0.6216**
SATISFACTION69	1.2684	2.1092	0.4976	0.5495
SIZE69	1.2489	2.3270	0.2234	0.6051

Number of cases = 13,606   Number of items = 16
Cronbach's alpha for the 16 questions = 0.6163

Table 9 shows how the alpha coefficient would change if any single question were deleted from the housing deprivation index for the 1969 sweep. There are three variables which, if removed from the index, would increase reliability marginally. These are:

- Mother of cohort member unsatisfied with ownership (for example, 'our home') of accommodation.

- Mother of cohort member unsatisfied with other aspects of accommodation.

- Mother of cohort member unsatisfied with location of accommodation.

The largest increase in Cronbach's alpha is achieved by removing 'Mother of cohort member unsatisfied with ownership (for example, "our home") of accommodation' from the housing deprivation index. This variable is also not associated with a significant increased risk of 'poor' health (see Appendix C, Table 23) and so it has been omitted from the final index. By contrast, the most statistically reliable measure of housing deprivation was the cohort member's mother's 'subjective' satisfaction with the accommodation. The final housing deprivation index for the 1969 sweep of the NCDS has a Cronbach's alpha of 0.6216.

Housing deprivation in 1974

Logistic regression models were estimated for each of the 10 variables in the 1974 sweep of the NCDS that could potentially be used as part of a housing deprivation index. The variables are:

- Cohort member has to share a bed with others.

- Living in a flat.

- Overcrowding (more than one person per room).

- Front door of the accommodation on or above the third floor of the building.

- Not having sole access to hot water.

- Not having sole access to a bath.

- Not having a room to do homework, etc on your own in the accommodation.

- Living in non-self-contained accommodation (rooms, caravans, etc).

- Lacking or having to share an indoor toilet.

- Not having sole access to a cooker.

Summary tables for the analysis are presented in Appendix C (Tables 26-35). Unfortunately, there were no questions in the 1974 sweep on either the cohort member's or their parents' satisfaction with the accommodation. However, a number of the housing deprivation variables that had been asked in previous sweeps had, by 1974, become highly significant predictors of 'poor' health. For example, the most statistically significant variable is whether the cohort member has to share a bed with others (Appendix C, Table 26), which had not been such a highly 'significant' variable in previous sweeps. This illustrates the relative nature of housing deprivation: while it might be considered appropriate (or even fun) for 7-year-old children to share a bedroom or even a bed, it represents a severe housing deprivation for a 16-year-old to have to do so. The 1983 *Breadline Britain* survey (Mack and Lansley, 1985) showed that 77% of a representative sample of the British population considered that it was 'necessary' for every child over 10 of separate sexes to have their own bedroom. All 10 variables are positively associated with an increased risk of 'poor' health. However, not having sole access to a cooker affected so few households by 1974 that it was not significant at the 5% level (Appendix C, Table 35).

Reliability analysis for housing deprivation variables at age 16

Table 10 summarises the reliability results for the 10 potential housing deprivation questions in the 1974 sweep of the NCDS. The overall Cronbach's coefficient alpha for the 16 questions is 0.4513, which is considerably less than the 0.70 level that is desirable. The housing deprivation questions in the 1974 sweep are clearly far less reliable than those in the two previous sweeps. This is almost certainly because by 1974 questions concerned with the lack of basic amenities, overcrowding and tenure were insensitive indicators of housing deprivation. The relatively low Cronbach's alpha indicates that households that suffered from one type of housing deprivation (for example, overcrowding) were relatively unlikely to also suffer from a lack of basic amenities. The 'housing' deprivation variables in the 1974 sweep therefore cannot be combined into a very reliable index.

Table 10 shows how the alpha coefficient would change if any single question was deleted from the housing deprivation index from the 1974 sweep. The only question that would increase alpha if it were omitted was not having sole access to a cooker. This variable is also not associated with a significant increased risk of 'poor' health (see Appendix C, Table 35) and so it has been omitted from the final index. The final housing deprivation index for the 1974 sweep of the NCDS has a Cronbach's alpha of 0.4544.

Table 10: Reliability of the 10 housing deprivation questions: 1974 sweep

Variable	Scale mean if item deleted	Scale variance if item deleted	Corrected item – total correlation	Alpha if item deleted
BATH74	0.7023	0.8404	0.3577	0.3794
BED74	0.6588	0.8199	0.2103	0.4137
COOK74	**0.7360**	**0.9887**	**0.0636**	**0.4544**
CROWD16	0.3905	0.5840	0.2531	0.4235
FLATS74	0.6534	0.8532	0.1261	0.4475
HIRISE74	0.7212	0.9456	0.1362	0.4410
HOTW74	0.7086	0.8678	0.3182	0.3954
HWORK74	0.6454	0.8421	0.1303	0.4474
LAV74	0.6887	0.8366	0.2842	0.3929
NOTSELF74	0.7309	0.9700	0.1170	0.4472

Number of cases = 11,257   Number of items = 10
Cronbach's alpha for the 10 questions = 0.4513

Housing deprivation in 1981

Logistic regression models were estimated for each of the nine variables in the 1981 sweep of the NCDS that could potentially be used as part of a housing deprivation index. The variables are:

- Cohort member has been homeless.

- Dissatisfied with present accommodation.

- Front door of the accommodation on or above the third floor of the building.

- Living in non self-contained accommodation (rooms, caravans, etc).

- Overcrowding (more than one person per room).

- Not having sole access to a bath.

- Lacking or having to share an indoor toilet.

- Not having sole access to a kitchen.

- Accommodation is below the 'bedroom' standard.

Summary tables for the analysis are presented in Appendix C, Tables 36-44. The most statistically significant predictor of 'poor' health at age 23 was whether the cohort member had been homeless by this age. This supports the findings of many previous studies on the serious and long-term health consequences of homelessness. The only other variable that was associated with 'poor' health at less than the 5% level of significance was the cohort member's satisfaction with their accommodation (Appendix C, Table 37). Although all the other variables on lack of basic amenities, tenure and overcrowding were positively associated with 'poor' health, none of them were significant at the 5% level. The least significant variable indicated whether the accommodation met the (1981) bedroom standard (Appendix C, Table 44).

These results provide a further illustration of both the 'relative' nature of housing deprivation to position in the life-course and the increasing irrelevance of 'basic amenities'-type questions as adequate measures of deprivation by the 1980s. By 1981 many cohort members had left their parental homes and were living in 'student'-type accommodation; for example, they had not yet formed their own separate households but were living with unrelated friends. What constitutes housing deprivation for a family with young children – such as living in a high rise flat without an adequate lift or having to share facilities with others – may represent only a minor inconvenience for a fit young adult of 23.

Reliability analysis for housing deprivation variables at age 23

Table 11 shows the summary reliability results for the nine potential housing deprivation questions in the 1981 sweep of the NCDS. The overall Cronbach's coefficient alpha for the 16 questions is 0.4732, which is considerably less than the 0.70 level that is desirable. The housing deprivation questions in the 1981 sweep of the NCDS are far less reliable than those in the 1965 and 1969 sweeps. The level of reliability had not, however, deteriorated since 1974, although the nature of the problem causing the unreliability may have changed. The low level of reliability by 1981 is almost certainly because the 'housing deprivation' questions were not particularly appropriate to the life-course stage of the cohort members. The relatively low Cronbach's alpha indicates that households that suffered from one type of housing deprivation (for example, overcrowding) were relatively unlikely to also suffer from a lack of basic amenities. The 'housing' deprivation variables in the 1981 sweep therefore cannot be combined into a very reliable index.

Table 11 shows how the alpha coefficient would change if any single question was deleted from the housing deprivation index from the 1981 sweep. Alpha would increase if four of the nine questions were omitted. These were:

- Cohort member has been homeless.
- Dissatisfied with present accommodation.
- Front door of the accommodation on or above the third floor of the building.
- Accommodation is below the 'bedroom' standard.

However, homelessness and the cohort member's satisfaction with their accommodation were the only two variables that were significantly associated with an increased risk of 'poor' health. The variable with the least association with the risk of 'poor' health was the 'bedroom standard' (see Appendix C, Table 44) and so it has been omitted from the final index.

The final housing deprivation index for the 1981 sweep of the NCDS has a Cronbach's alpha of 0.4842. However, it must be noted that the housing deprivation index for the fourth sweep (1981) of the NCDS cannot be considered to be either very reliable or valid. The wrong questions were asked to measure housing deprivation at this point in the cohort member's life-course.

Table 11: Reliability of the nine housing deprivation questions: 1981 sweep

Variable	Scale mean if item deleted	Corrected variance if item deleted	Item – total correlation	Alpha if item deleted
BATH81	0.3593	0.4908	0.4715	0.3661
COOK81	0.3603	0.4991	0.4432	0.3768
CROWD23	0.3506	0.5215	0.2450	0.4297
HIRISE81	**0.3679**	**0.5977**	**0.0195**	**0.4891**
HOMELESS81	**0.3280**	**0.5522**	**0.0358**	**0.5119**
LAV81	0.3414	0.4766	0.3586	0.3830
NOTSELF81	0.3772	0.5755	0.2840	0.4459
SATISFIED81	0.3274	0.5336	0.0898	0.4911
BEDSTAND81	**0.2587**	**0.4304**	**0.1778**	**0.4842**

Number of cases = 11,752   Number of items = 9
Cronbach's alpha for the 9 questions = 0.4732

Housing deprivation in 1991

Logistic regression models were estimated for each of the 10 variables in the 1991 sweep of the NCDS that could potentially be used as part of a housing deprivation index. The variables are:

- Cohort member has been homeless.
- Dissatisfied with the area they live in.
- Dissatisfied with present accommodation.
- Accommodation has had serious problems of damp or mould.
- Overcrowding (more than one person per room).
- Front door of the accommodation on or above the third floor of the building.
- Living in non-self-contained accommodation (rooms, caravans, etc).
- Not having sole access to a bath.
- Not having sole access to a kitchen.
- Lacking or having to share an indoor toilet.

The results are summarised in Appendix C, Tables 45-54. The most statistically significant predictors of 'poor' health were whether the cohort member had been homeless (Appendix C, Table 45) and their satisfaction with their area and accommodation (Appendix C, Tables 46 and 47 respectively). The only other two variables that were significantly associated with 'poor' health at the less than the 5% level of significance were if the accommodation had suffered from serious problems of damp or mould (Appendix C, Table 48) and if it was overcrowded (Appendix C, Table 49). By 1991 when the cohort members were 33, most of them had formed their own households and had their own families. Questions on overcrowding had again become appropriate to their life-course stage. However, by 1991 questions concerning the lack of basic amenities were devoid of any predictive power.

Reliability analysis for housing deprivation variables at age 33

Table 12 shows the summary reliability results for the 10 potential housing deprivation questions in the 1991 sweep of the NCDS. The overall Cronbach's coefficient alpha for the 16 questions is an extremely low 0.3116, which is considerably less than half the 0.70 level that is desirable. The housing deprivation questions in the 1991 sweep are far less reliable than those in all the previous sweeps. This is almost certainly because by 1991 questions concerned with the lack of basic amenities were inappropriate indicators of housing deprivation. The relatively low Cronbach's alpha indicates that households that suffered from one type of housing deprivation (for example, overcrowding) were very unlikely to also suffer from lack of a basic amenity. The 'housing' deprivation variables in the 1991 sweep therefore cannot be combined into a reliable index.

Table 12 shows how the alpha coefficient would change if any single question were deleted from the housing deprivation index from the 1991 sweep. The only question that would increase alpha if it were omitted is 'overcrowding'. This variable was one of the five that was associated with a significant increased risk of 'poor' health (see Appendix C, Table 49) and so it has not been omitted from the final index. The final housing deprivation index for the 1991 sweep of the NCDS has a Cronbach's alpha of 0.3116. The index is valid but it is unreliable.

Table 12: Reliability of the 10 housing deprivation questions: 1991 sweep

Variable	Scale mean if item deleted	Corrected variance if item deleted	Item – total correlation	Alpha if item deleted
AREA91	0.3519	0.4042	0.1906	0.2417
BATH91	0.4253	0.5272	0.1387	0.3033
COOK91	0.4250	0.5302	0.0788	0.3086
CROWD33	**0.3029**	**0.3848**	**0.1075**	**0.3121**
DAMP91	0.3051	0.3772	0.1327	0.2906
HIRISE91	0.4219	0.5252	0.0693	0.3074
HOME91	0.3897	0.4759	0.0982	0.2956
LAV91	0.4259	0.5295	0.1356	0.3056
NOTSEL91	0.4227	0.5243	0.0932	0.3043
SAT91	0.3734	0.4091	0.2694	0.2009

Number of cases = 9,848   Number of items = 10
Cronbach's alpha for the 10 questions = 0.3116

The reliability of the housing deprivation index

The foregoing analysis indicates that, while it is possible to construct housing deprivation indices on the basis of the NCDS data, the result is not as reliable as might be desirable. Clearly this has implications for the robustness of analysis which is based upon the index. The remainder of the analysis in this report needs to be interpreted in the light of this issue.

Yet it is important to put the results reported here in perspective. The housing deprivation variables in the NCDS are the same as those that have been used in virtually all other non-housing specific social surveys and censuses over the past 30 years. In fact the NCDS housing deprivation variables are probably better than those in most other general surveys. While the reliability of the housing deprivation indices are lower – much lower in later sweeps – than is desirable, their reliability is still much greater than that of many widely used deprivation indices such as the DOE Z Score, the Index of Local Conditions, and the Townsend Index (see Lee et al, 1995 for a critical discussion). Furthermore, although the housing deprivation indices have reliability problems, their validity is somewhat better.

At a broader level, the varying reliability of the housing deprivation indices is in itself an important finding. The commonly used indicators of housing deprivation are much more reliable and valid measures for families with children than for young single adult households. Our analysis points to the need to reconsider the indicators that we use to measure housing deprivation and to examine the possibility of developing alternative indicators that are capable of reliably capturing the housing deprivation experienced by different types of household. Appendix E gives details of a number of alternative housing and area deprivation indicators that have been used in other surveys. A number of these indicators represent alternative means of gathering information on respondents' subjective assessment of their neighbourhood and dwelling, which appear to be particularly valuable in construction of a reliable index. Importantly, these indicators are presented to illustrate how other surveys have approached the question of housing deprivation: whether their use would, in actuality, result in a more robust measure of housing deprivation than those questions already used by the NCDS is something which can only be determined through empirical research.

Housing deprivation index scores for the five sweeps

In examining housing deprivation across the five sweeps of the NCDS it is important to begin by reflecting upon two points. Firstly, as social expectations and standards improve over time, conditions which were once seen as perfectly acceptable become 'deprived' and consequently a problem that needs to be addressed. Yet, where a factor is considered as a candidate for inclusion in a housing deprivation index at all points in time, it is desirable to treat it as consistently as possible. As a result, where standards are set from a current perspective, this can have the effect of increasing apparent levels of deprivation in the past. Whether analysts addressing the question at the relevant point in the past would have accepted that the problem was quite such a large one is a different question.

Secondly, the method that we have used to construct the deprivation index makes maximum use of the data available in each sweep in an attempt to derive the most reliable index possible. As can be seen from Table 13, the differing availability of data

coupled with the changing importance of the available variables in measuring deprivation means that the maximum score possible on the index varies. An alternative approach to the problem is to include only those variables that are available across all the sweeps. While this would produce more consistency in the index, it would most likely lead to an index which was rendered irrelevant because of its increasing unreliability, as the results presented above suggest. The meaning and nature of deprivation changes over time and hence the most appropriate components for a deprivation index need to change over time if the index is to capture the phenomenon reliably.

Table 13 shows the distribution of the housing deprivation index for the five sweeps of the NCDS. In 1965 just over half of all households (51%) suffered at least one housing deprivation. The percentage of cohort members suffering from some housing deprivation rose between 1965 and 1969 and then declined to a minimum in 1981 when only a fifth (20%) of cohort members suffered from housing deprivation. However, by 1991, when most cohort members had formed their own families, the level of housing deprivation had increased to affect just less than a third (32%) of cohort members.

Table 13: Housing deprivation index score for the five sweeps of the NCDS

Housing deprivation index score	1965 %	1969 %	1974 %	1981 %	1991 %
0	48.8	44.7	60.6	79.8	67.9
1	30.6	22.5	24.5	14.9	23.1
2	9.2	14.9	10.1	1.8	6.2
3	4.3	7.9	3.2	1.6	1.8
4	2.8	5.0	1.0	1.4	0.7
5	2.2	2.4	0.4	0.4	0.2
6	1.3	1.2	0.1	0.1	–
7	0.6	0.8	–	–	–
8	0.1	0.3	–	–	–
9	–	0.2	–	–	–
10	–	0.1	–	–	–
Total	100.0	100.0	100.0	100.0	100.0

Table 14 shows the number of times that cohort members had suffered from at least one housing deprivation in their lives. Twenty-two per cent of cohort members who were included in the 1965 sweep of the NCDS had never suffered from any housing deprivation by the time they were 33. Conversely, 1.4% of cohort members had been living in 'poor' housing conditions in each sweep of the NCDS.

Table 14: Number of sweeps that cohort members who were present in NCDS sweep 1 had suffered from any housing deprivation

Number of times	Number of cases	% suffering housing deprivation
Never	3,387	22.0
Once	3,930	25.5
Twice	3,696	24.0
Three times	3,058	19.8
Four times	1,145	7.4
Five times	209	1.4
Total	15,425	100.0

Note: All cohort members present in sweep 1 are included in this table.

Table 15 shows the number of times that cohort members had suffered from multiple (that is, at least two) housing deprivation in their lives. Fifty-three per cent of cohort members who were included in the 1965 sweep of the NCDS had never suffered from multiple housing deprivation by the time they were 33. Conversely, 0.6% of cohort members had been suffering from multiple housing deprivation during four out of the five NCDS sweeps.

Housing deprivation over the life-course

In order to explore the impact of housing deprivation over the life-course upon ill-health, a pathways analysis was undertaken. Figures 8(a) and 8(b) illustrate the pathways of housing deprivation experienced by the NCDS cohort members. For the purposes of this analysis, housing deprivation is defined as a score of one or more on the housing deprivation index (see Table 13). The pathways analysis starts with housing deprivation at the age of 7 because of the limited housing variables available on the 1958 sweep.

Table 15: Number of sweeps that cohort members who were present in NCDS sweep 1 have suffered from multiple housing deprivation (for example, with a housing deprivation index score of two or more)

Number of times	Number of cases	% suffering multiple housing deprivation
Never	8,240	53.4
Once	4,231	27.4
Twice	2,109	13.7
Three times	746	4.8
Four times	92	0.6
Five times	7	0.0
Total	15,425	100.0

Note: All cohort members present in sweep 1 are included in this table.

Despite over half of the cohort members living in circumstances of housing deprivation at age 7, the pathways analysis shows that only a small proportion of the cohort experienced housing deprivation throughout their life-course to the age of 33 (3%). The pathways analysis of housing deprivation indicates that entry into circumstances of housing deprivation from a situation of non-deprivation is not common. In contrast, most of those experiencing housing deprivation at age 7 were still experiencing housing deprivation at age 11 and many continued to do so at age 16. Thus nearly a quarter of the cohort experienced housing deprivation during each of the three childhood sweeps (ages 7, 11, 16). In most other cases the majority of those who find themselves in a situation of housing deprivation in one sweep moved to a position of no deprivation in the next.

In assessing the impact of housing deprivation over the life-course upon ill-health, odds ratios were calculated using a dichotomous version of the severity of ill-health index as described above. The results are presented in Figures 9(a) and 9(b).

In childhood the highest odds ratios are recorded by cohort members who had experienced housing deprivation at age 11 (1.42), regardless of whether or not they had experienced housing deprivation at age 7. In sweep 3 cohort members whose pathways include deprivation at age 16 recorded considerably higher odds of experiencing moderate or severe health problems at 16 than those following other pathways. And it is those who had also experienced housing deprivation at 11 who recorded the highest risk of experiencing ill-health, whether they experienced housing deprivation at age 7 (odds ratio of 1.71) or not (odds ratio of 1.82). The likelihood of those cohort members who experienced housing deprivation at age 7 and 16, but not 11, experiencing ill-health was similar to that of those who only experienced deprivation at 16 (1.49 and 1.40 respectively). Those cohort members who only experienced housing deprivation at the age of 7 (1.00) and those who had only experienced housing deprivation at age 11 recorded an odds ratio (1.03) not significantly different from 1.0.

By the time we move to sweep 4 of the NCDS we start encountering pathways which are being followed by few cohort members. All the pathways which entail cohort members experiencing housing deprivation at age 23 and contain more than 20 observations at age 23 record odds ratios greater than one, although in two cases the odds ratio is not substantially different from 1.00. A first experience of housing deprivation at 23 does not appear to increase the risk of ill-health substantially. At the other extreme, those who had experienced some degree of housing deprivation at all sweeps of the NCDS did not record substantially greater odds of experiencing ill-health at 23 than those who had less extensive experience of deprivation. Indeed those who did not experience deprivation until age 16 but who continued in deprived circumstances at age 23 recorded the highest odds of suffering health problems (odds ratio of 1.99).

Most of the pathways which entail cohort members living in non-deprived housing circumstances at age 23 record odds ratios of less than one at age 23. This suggests that such groups, although they may have experienced deprivation at some point in the past, are less likely to be ill at 23 than those who have never experienced deprivation. The only exception is those who experienced deprivation at 7 and 11 but who have subsequently lived in non-deprived housing circumstances (odds ratio of 1.23).

In relation to the sweep 5 we observe most of those currently living in circumstances of housing deprivation having odds ratios greater than one, although in some cases only marginally greater. The picture for those who were not living in circumstances of housing deprivation in 1991 is less clear cut in as much as some recorded odds ratios above one while others recorded odds ratios below one. The highest odds ratio (1.72) for a pathway with more than 20 observations at age 33 was recorded among the small number who had experienced deprivation at every point on the pathway, with those who experienced housing deprivation at every point until 23 but not at 33 also having a substantially heightened likelihood of ill-health (1.41). Interestingly, the two other pathways which record a notably heightened likelihood of ill-health at 33 are those who were experiencing housing deprivation at age 33 and had also experienced housing deprivation at age 16.

A number of possible competing interpretations of the link between housing deprivation and ill-health could be offered. Figures 9(a) and 9(b) do not provide unambiguous support for any one particular interpretation. The simplest interpretation is that current housing circumstances are the main housing influence on ill-health and the figures certainly lend some support to a concern for current conditions. An alternative approach would be to look for an 'accumulation of risks' and expect to see those with consecutive experiences of housing deprivation exhibiting greater likelihood of ill-health than those with 'interrupted' experiences of housing deprivation. It is true that, with the exception of age 23, those who are deprived throughout show some of the larger odds ratios and also that some pathways which include consecutive experiences of housing deprivation seem to also exhibit relatively high ratios, but the pattern is by no means consistent. More importantly, an 'accumulation of risk' interpretation of the likelihood of ill-health should ideally not focus upon the impact of a single factor alone but should be equally concerned with the interaction between risk factors. A third interpretation is that it is experience in early childhood, coupled with current experience in

Figure 8(a): Housing deprivation pathway (%): deprived at age 7

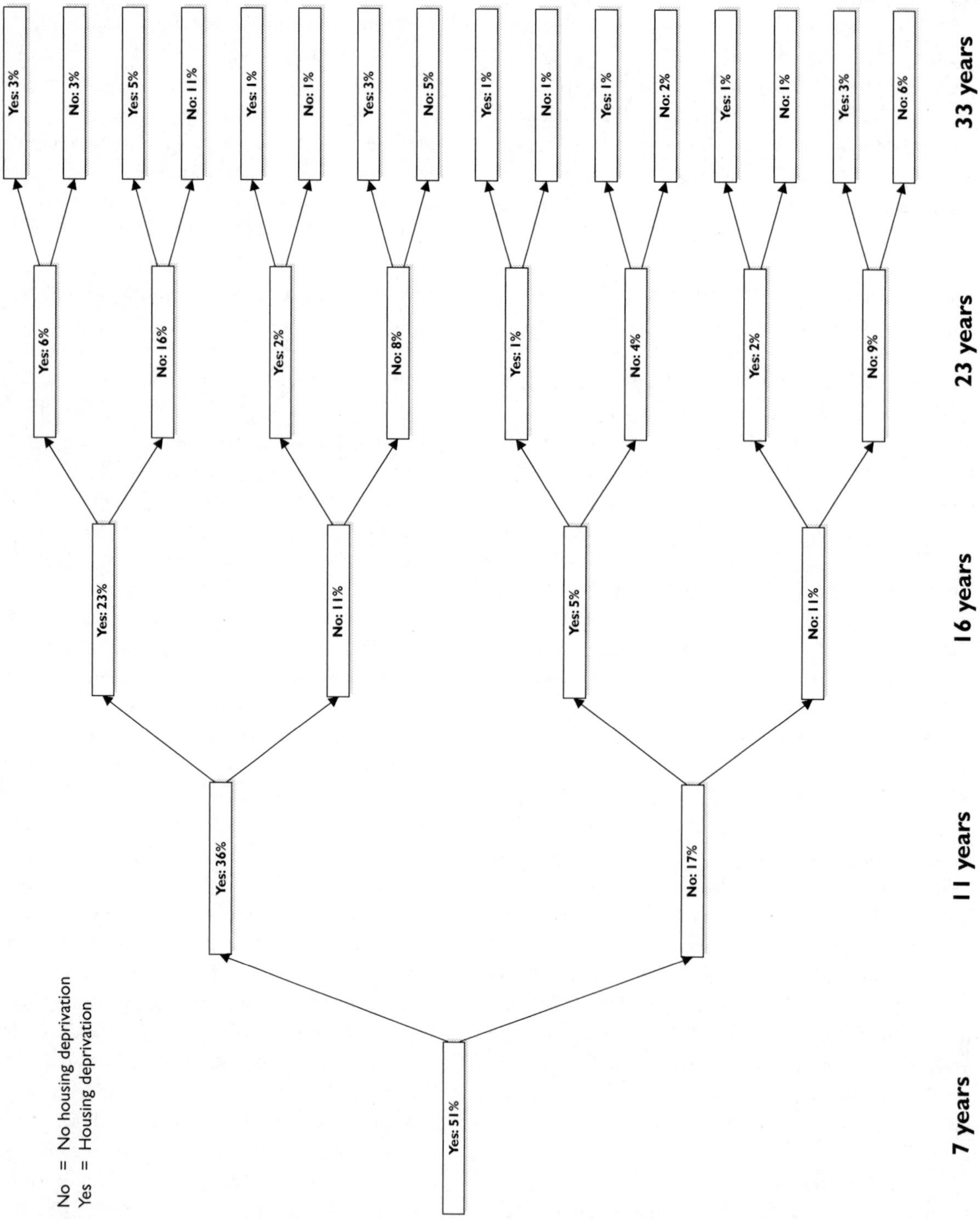

No = No housing deprivation
Yes = Housing deprivation

| 7 years | 11 years | 16 years | 23 years | 33 years |

Figure 8(b): Housing deprivation pathway (%): not deprived at age 7

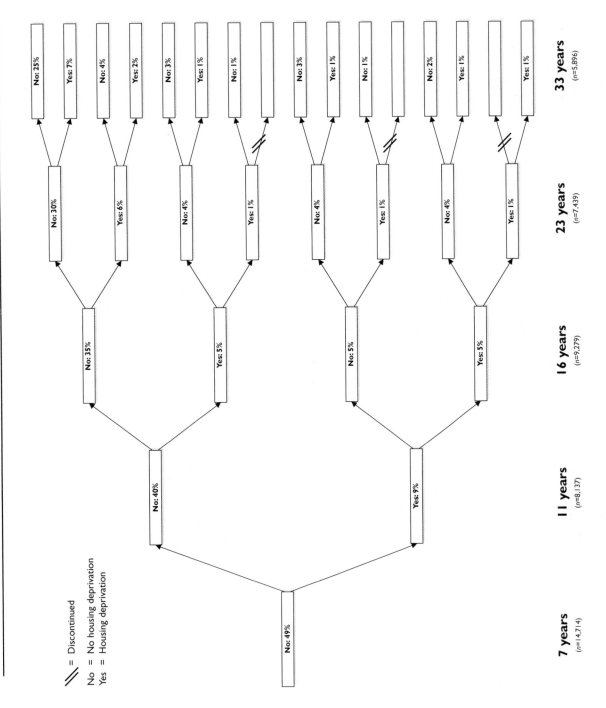

// = Discontinued

No = No housing deprivation
Yes = Housing deprivation

7 years
(n=14,714)

11 years
(n=8,137)

16 years
(n=9,279)

23 years
(n=7,439)

33 years
(n=5,896)

Figure 9(a): Severe or moderate health problems by housing deprivation pathway (odds ratio): deprived at age 7

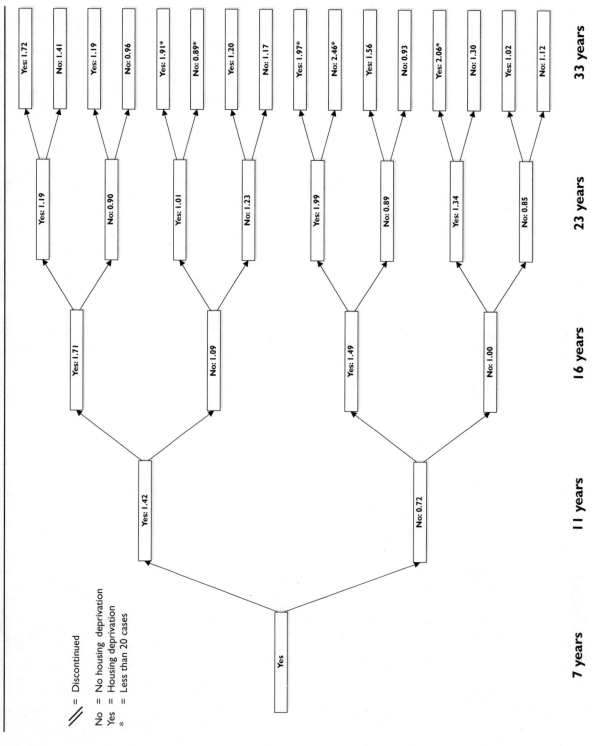

Figure 9(b): Severe or moderate health problems by housing deprivation pathway (odds ratio): not deprived at age 7

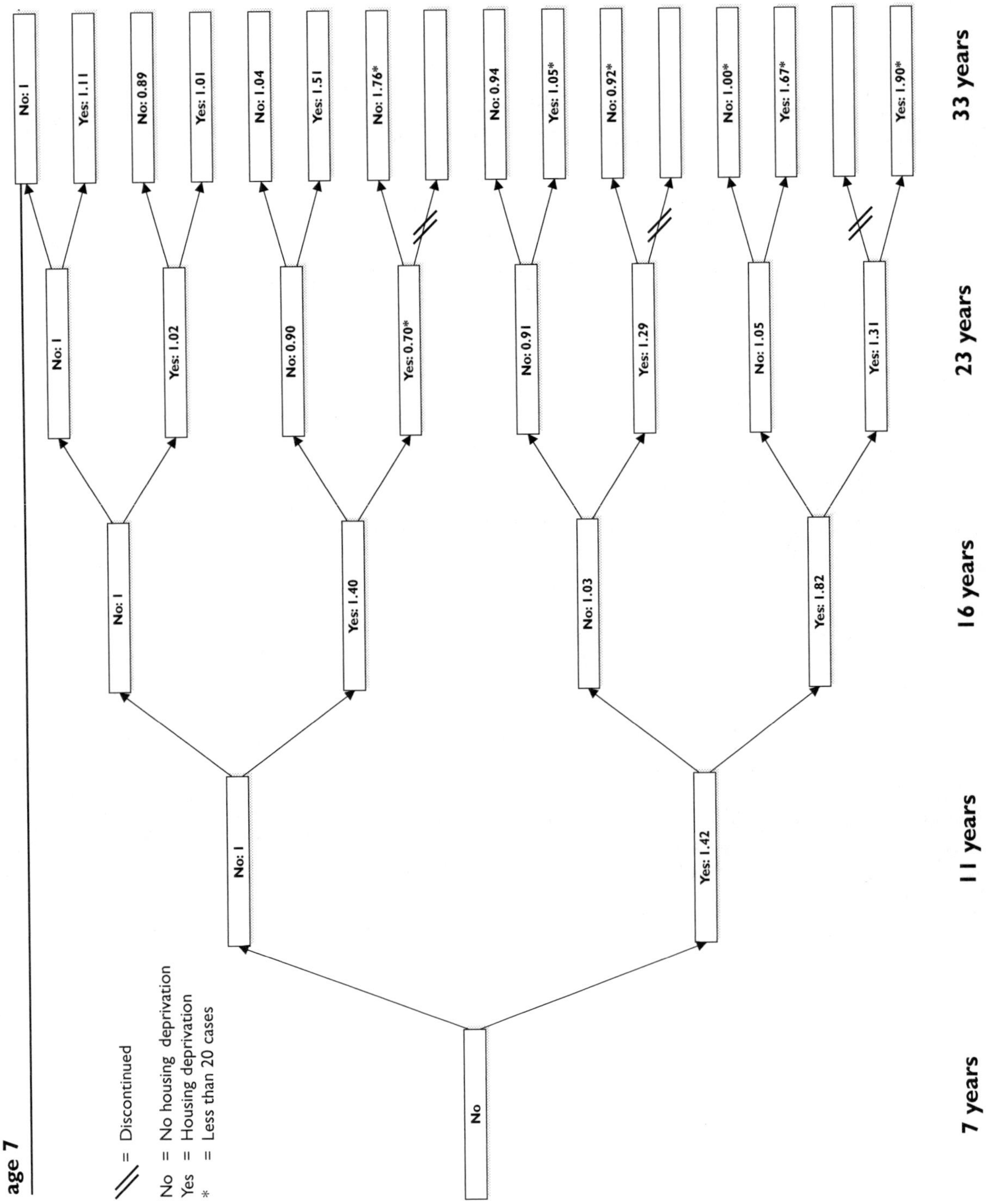

// = Discontinued

No = No housing deprivation
Yes = Housing deprivation
* = Less than 20 cases

7 years   11 years   16 years   23 years   33 years

Figure 10: Severe or moderate health problems by housing deprivation at the age of 33

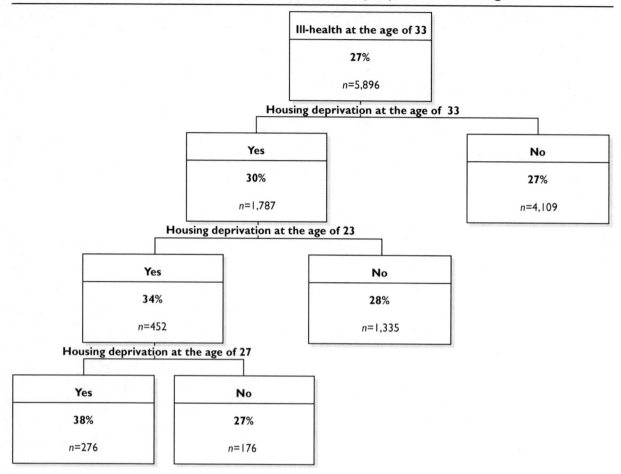

adult life, which is the key to understanding current health status. Assessing this interpretation is hampered by the relative lack of reliable odds ratios at age 33 in Figure 9(b) but, by inspection, it could be suggested that the odds ratios at age 33 tend to be higher in Figure 9(a) than those in Figure 9(b). Clearly this is no more than conjecture at this stage. A fourth interpretation takes a step back from the focus on early childhood to argue that there may be a 'critical period' in development during which the experience of housing deprivation has particularly damaging implications for health in adulthood. Investigation of such an interpretation requires a more sophisticated mode of analysis and it is therefore appropriate to investigate these data using CHAID (Figure 10).

Chi-squared automatic interaction detector analysis

A CHAID analysis was conducted to investigate the most statistically significant housing deprivation variables affecting ill-health at the age of 33. At the age of 33, 27% of NCDS cohort members suffered from severe or moderate ill-health. Current housing deprivation emerges as the most important factor affecting whether cohort members were likely to experience ill-health at the age of 33. Thirty per cent of those cohort members who experienced housing deprivation at the age of 33 suffered from ill-health. This group was further sub-divided by whether they had experienced housing deprivation at the age of 23. Thus, 34% of those subjects who had experienced housing deprivation at both 33 and 23 suffered ill-health at the age of 33. Furthermore, risks of ill-health were exacerbated for these subjects if they had also experienced housing deprivation at the age of 7. Thirty-eight per cent of subjects who had experienced housing deprivation throughout their adulthood and who had also experienced housing deprivation at 7 suffered from ill-health at the age of 33.

Thus, in an analysis focusing upon housing deprivation in isolation, CHAID suggests that the key influences upon ill-health are deprivation in adulthood and in early childhood. Although in itself not in any sense conclusive, the fact that the analysis did not identify housing deprivation in either the sweep at age 11 or 16 as statistically significant suggests that if there is a critical period in development during which housing deprivation affects health then it is indeed in early, rather than later, childhood.

Summary and reflection

From a life-course perspective this analysis, which focuses upon health and housing without attempting to incorporate other types of risk, does not provide any strong support for the proposition that an accumulation of housing risk throughout the life-course is a key consideration. Nonetheless, our analysis suggests that the role that housing deprivation might play in causing moderate or severe ill-health is likely to be focused on conditions in adulthood and early childhood. This is in accord with much of the existing literature, but rather than assuming the case the analysis examined and rejected housing deprivation in the intervening period as a statistically significant factor in determining health in adulthood.

Our attempt to create a housing deprivation index to be used across all sweeps of the NCDS met with mixed success. The variables included in the indices were strongly associated with ill-health, but it became clear that although the sort of housing-related questions which were asked on the NCDS had great relevance in the 1960s, this relevance declined rapidly, such that for the later sweeps, unreliable indices were being generated.

This decline in relevance can be interpreted at two levels. On the one hand, reflecting upon three decades of housing policy it is clear that much has changed. As a result of new housing investment, tenure change and falling family size, many of the original indicators of housing deprivation – especially concern with basic amenities – have become increasingly redundant. The growth of public renting built to Parker Morris standards in particular has contributed to a dramatic increase in amenity standards. As lack of amenities and overcrowding have declined in significance since the 1970s, concerns about housing deprivation shifted towards the coincidence of poverty and unfitness and disrepair (strongly associated with low-income home ownership and private renting) and the more general association between concentrated poverty and the less desirable parts of the council sector. Over the life of the NCDS, therefore, the links between bad housing, poverty and ill-health have become more complex. Broadly stated, the worst physical conditions are now to be found in the private sector but the vast majority of the poor are living in council housing, a tenure with relatively high levels of amenity provision. A separate, but not necessarily alternative, interpretation would focus upon cohort effects and note that it may be that specific housing indicators are not sensitive enough to identify housing deprivation at particular life-cycle stages. So, for example, while overcrowding may be an indication of housing deprivation during late childhood or the early stages of parenthood it may not in itself represent a problem among young single adults.

We would suggest that there is a pressing need for the DETR to provide guidance on a set of new sensitive housing deprivation indicators that are suitable for use in general government and other social surveys such as the NCDS. These new indicators of housing deprivation are conspicuous by their absence from the current Office for National Statistics (ONS) harmonisation proposals. However, potentially suitable questions are available in the Survey of English Housing, the English Housing Conditions Survey and the European Household Panel Survey (see Appendix D for details of possible questions).

6

A longitudinal analysis of the impact of housing upon health

In this chapter we place housing deprivation in the context of other factors which can influence health. The first part focuses upon the circumstances of cohort members in 1991 and the second part goes on to present a longitudinal analysis which attempts to disentangle the effect of housing deprivation upon health from the effect of the range of other factors.

The effects of housing deprivation on morbidity after allowing for other causes of ill-health

The previous chapter showed the strong association between various measures of housing deprivation and 'poor' health across the NCDS cohort members' life-course. However, there are many other factors that have been shown to cause ill-health. The range of factors is summarised in Figure 11 which groups them into six categories: standard of living, behaviour, housing, social, environment and genetic. Each of these groupings contains a number of subcategories of factors that have been causally linked to health outcomes. For example, the genetic category contains birth weight, age, heredity, and gender, all of which can and do influence health.

The purpose of this chapter is to discover if housing deprivation has an independent effect on health after allowing for all the other factors that also affect a cohort member's health outcome. It should be noted from Figure 11 that several factors that are commonly used in health studies (such as social class

and tenure) have not been included in the model. Although social class and tenure are associated with 'poor' health, they do not in themselves cause ill-health, rather they act as proxies for a range of more specific factors which are not modelled explicitly. Because the NCDS offers the opportunity to examine these more specific factors directly to include the proxy variables as well would result in misspecification.

The multivariate analysis began with the 23 variables described in Table 16. Most of the variables are based on individual questions in the NCDS, rather than being derived. So, for example, a cohort member reporting that she or he was dissatisfied with current accommodation would be given a score of one on this variable and those who did not indicate dissatisfaction were scored zero.

These 23 variables encompass many (but not all) the factors in Figure 11. The NCDS contains a wealth of information but it is a general survey and so it does not contain information on all possible factors which could cause ill-health. For example, there is no information on Radon levels or pollution. There is little information on ethnicity or whether the cohort member has suffered from prejudice: these factors have been inferred from the country of birth of the cohort member and their parents. It has been assumed that if this is recorded as Africa, the Indian subcontinent or the Caribbean then the cohort member is more likely to have suffered from prejudice and discrimination which may have affected their health.

Figure 11: Factors influencing health

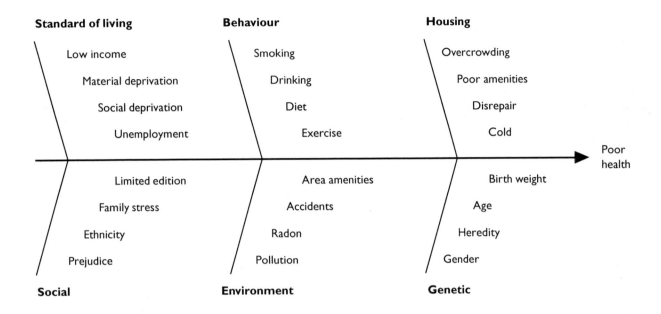

Table 16: Variables available for multivariate analysis of 1991 sweep

Variable	Description	Values/level of measurement
HOMELESS91	Cohort member has been homeless	Binary
SAT91	Dissatisfied with present accommodation	Binary
AREA91	Dissatisfied with the area they live in	Binary
DAMP91	Accommodation has had serious problems of damp or mould	Binary
CROWD91	Overcrowding (more than one person per room)	Binary
HIRISE91	Front door of the accommodation on or above the third floor of the building	Binary
NOTSELF91	Living in non-self-contained accommodation (rooms, caravans, etc)	Binary
BATH91	Not having sole access to a bath	Binary
COOK91	Not having sole access to a kitchen	Binary
LAV91	Lacking or having to share an indoor toilet	Binary
COB	Country of birth	Categorical
N622	Sex of cohort member	Binary
N516	Birthweight of cohort member	Continuous
CONGEN	Congenital disease	Binary
DEATH	Death of spouse or own child	Binary
DIVORCE	Divorce of cohort member	Binary
N2397	Age mother figure left full-time education	Continuous
UNEMP*	Unemployment of cohort member	Binary
FINANCE*	Serious financial problems	Binary
SMOKE	Cigarettes smoked per day	Continuous
DRINK	How often cohort member drinks alcohol	Interval
ACTIV33	Amount of exercise	Interval
DEBT33	Financial problems and debts	Binary

Note: Variables UNEMP and FINANCE were included as proxies for low income as clean income data is currently not available for all five sweeps of the NCDS.

Perhaps the central concern for policy is whether housing deprivation has an effect upon health independent of the effects of low income. In order to examine this question fully it is desirable to have robust data on income levels. Yet, as Table 16 indicates, the information on income which the NCDS offers cannot readily be employed in analysis. Our research relied on 'experience of unemployment' and 'serious financial problems' as alternative, and less satisfactory, indicators of low income levels. It is regrettable that an income variable is not available, but we believe that the available variables allow us to incorporate indicators of low 'standard of living' into the analysis and that it is low standard of living rather than low income per se which is likely to be deleterious.

Table 17 shows the summary results from a stepwise logistic regression analysis of the health of cohort members in the 1991 sweep of the NCDS. The results are from a binary logistic regression with the health index dichotomised into 'disabled/severe and moderate' ill-health versus 'minor or no' health problems. The analysis employed a backwards elimination procedure using the likelihood ratio as the selection criterion.

Table 17 shows that out of the original 23 variables entered into the stepwise logistic regression model, 10 are significant in the final model. The right hand column 'Significance' indicates the level of statistical significance that the variable achieved. The conventional critical value for making statistical judgements is 0.050 which indicates that there is only a one in 20 (that is, 5%) chance that the estimated coefficient is a product of chance rather than a genuine association. It can be seen that all the variables in Table 17 achieve this value except 'divorce', which is slightly outside it. It can also be seen that many of the variables have significance levels very much below 5% which means that the probability of these associations being a product of chance is correspondingly smaller.

The most statistically significant factors are 'genetic' (sex and congenital ill-health), 'behavioural' (drinking and smoking) and 'standard of living' (financial hardship and debts). Social factors such as the family stress caused by divorce are also important. Yet, after allowing for all these other factors housing deprivation factors still have a highly significant impact upon health. The three statistically significant housing deprivation factors were:

- Homeless – cohort member has been homeless
- Area91 – dissatisfied with the area they live in
- Notself91 – living in non self-contained accommodation (rooms, caravans, etc)

Table 17: Stepwise binary logistic regression results for the most significant variables that cause 'poor' health in the 1991 sweep of the NCDS

Variable	Odds ratio	95% confidence interval	Significance
AREA91	1.36	1.08-1.71	0.009
HOMELESS	1.44	1.06-1.96	0.021
NOTSELF91	4.22	1.18-15.10	0.027
CONGEN	1.15	1.06-1.24	0.000
SEX	1.24	1.09-1.40	0.001
DRINK	1.10	1.04-1.17	0.001
DEBT33	1.36	1.11-1.66	0.002
SMOKE	1.08	1.01-1.16	0.016
UNEM33	1.38	1.02-1.86	0.036
DIVORCE	1.10	0.99-1.22	0.066

Beyond the issue of statistical significance is the issue of substantive significance or importance: a variable can be statistically significant without being important in the sense of having a substantial effect in practice. From Table 17 it can be seen that the housing variables in the model are not only statistically significant but also substantively significant. The odds ratio for the increased risk of severe/moderate ill-health caused by past homelessness increased to 1.44 after allowing for the effects of the other variables in the model. The analysis thus indicates that past homelessness led to a 44% (on average) greater risk of severe/moderate ill-health of the NCDS cohort members in 1991. Similarly, dissatisfaction with the area was associated with a 36% (on average) greater risk of severe/moderate ill-health.

Because we do not have data from all members of the relevant population these figures are estimates of the true value of the odds ratios. A confidence interval (CI) is calculated to indicate the range within which the true value of the odds ratio will lie. A 95% CI indicates the range within which the true value will lie on 19 out of 20 occasions: on 5% of occasions the true value will lie outside of this range. Table 17 shows therefore that the true effect for the 'homeless' variable lies between increasing risk by 8% and increasing risk by 71%, with a one in 20 – that is relatively small – chance that it lies outside this range. Thus, even at the lower end of this range the analysis indicates an effect that is important in reality, and the chances of this effect being a statistical artifact are relatively small. It is also clear from the table that the variable NOTSELF91 seems to have a very substantial effect upon the risk of severe/moderate ill-health, but that this effect is much less accurately estimated. While the effect of this variable is substantial, it is important to recognise that it is quantitatively less important than other effects identified because only a very small proportion of cohort members were living in non-self-contained accommodation in 1991.

It is clear that after controlling for the other factors that can cause ill-health, housing deprivation emerges as an independent cause of 'poor' health among the cohort members in 1991. This result confirms the results of previous studies discussed in Chapter 2. However, a static cross-sectional analysis from one sweep cannot show the relationships between the duration and intensity of housing deprivation and 'poor' health over time. This requires a full longitudinal analysis.

The longitudinal effects of housing deprivation on morbidity

During the five sweeps of the NCDS a significant number of the original cohort members were not traced. They have disappeared from the survey and are technically considered to be 'censored' cases, that is, they have gone missing and it is not known what happened to them. Logistic regression is not a suitable technique to study data longitudinally when censored cases are present. The most widely used method for the longitudinal analysis of data of this nature is Cox's proportional hazard regression modelling. Cox's regression allows the analysis of time-to-event data in the presence of censored cases. Cox's regression requires relatively few assumptions

about the nature of the data, observations should be independent and the hazard ratio should be constant over time. That is, the proportionality of hazards from one case to another should not vary with time.

This proportionate hazards assumption is likely to be correct for variables that do not change over time, for example, the sex of the cohort member. Such variables can be thought of as attributes of the individual. However, many of the key variables that are causally related to ill-health vary with time. For example, the employment status of the cohort member's father figure or of the cohort member themselves in adulthood clearly changes with time. The value of the unemployment status variable will be different on different sweeps of the NCDS. In order to incorporate variables of this nature, which violate the proportionate hazards assumption, an extended version of Cox's regression must be used which allows the specification of variables that vary over time (these are referred to technically as segmented time-dependent covariates).

Thus, the extended Cox's regression model allows one to examine the aggregated impact of various factors that are causally related to severe ill-health across the life-course. These models allow the simultaneous assessment of the effects of both variables that do not change with time (that is, attributes such as sex) as well as variables that do vary with time (such as unemployment). The Cox's models produce valid estimates of the effects of both individual independent variables and combinations of variables on the likelihood of suffering from severe ill-health across the life-course. However, the method is computationally demanding. With 12 variables and 5 time periods there are over 2,000 million possible interactions involved. In order to ensure that the analysis is tractable it is therefore necessary to restrict the number of independent variables entering the model.

The 12 variables that were included in the initial model are shown in Table 18. These variables were selected in an attempt to encompass the range of different factors that caused ill-health, as shown in Figure 11, while trying to minimise the amount of correlation between the variables. This is necessary when using many multivariate techniques which proceed by 'partitioning the variance' (or odds). If

two variables that have a considerable degree of
overlap (that is, they are highly correlated and are
effectively measuring the same thing) are entered
into a model, then the apparent significance of both
variables will be reduced.

Table 18: Variables available for longitudinal analysis of sweeps 1 to 5

Variable	Description	Values/level of measurement
HDEP	Housing deprivation index score	See text
COB	Country of birth	Categorical
N622	Sex of cohort member	Binary
N516	Birthweight of cohort member	Continuous
CONGEN	Congenital disease	Binary
DEATH	Death of a parent, sibling, spouse or own child	Binary
DIVORCE	Divorce of parents or cohort member	Binary
N2397	Age mother figure left full-time education	Continuous
UNEMP	Unemployment of father figure or cohort member	Binary
FINANCE	Serious financial problems	Binary
SMOKE	Cohort member smokes	Binary
DRINK	Cohort member frequently drinks alcohol	Binary

In order to determine the longitudinal effects of
housing deprivation on ill-health after allowing for
other relevant causal factors, a multivariate stepwise
Cox's regression model was constructed which
included both multiple time invariant and multiple
segmented time-dependent covariates. The
dependent variable for this analysis was the length of
time between birth and a cohort member's first
experience of disability or severe ill-health, as
defined by the health indices from sweeps 1 to 5 of
the NCDS. A backward elimination procedure,
using the likelihood ratio as the selection criterion,
was employed.

Performing the analysis with the dependent variable
as 'severe or moderate ill-health' would not produce
dramatically different results because the key
distinction is between cohort members with
moderate and 'some' ill-health, rather than between
those with moderate and those with severe ill-
health. It is analytically more convenient to focus
on those with severe ill-health. More importantly, it

is substantively appropriate because severe ill-health
places the most substantial demands upon individual,
social and health service resources.

Table 19 shows the summary results for the
significant results in the final stepwise Cox's
regression model. The cohort members' housing
deprivation index scores – lying between zero and a
maximum of 10 (see Chapter 5, Table 13) – for each
of sweeps 1 to 5 were included in this model. It is
clear that cohort members were at greater risk of
suffering from a disability or severe ill-health if they
were male, had a congenital illness, had suffered the
stress of their own divorce or their parents
divorcing, if they smoked or drank a lot of alcohol
or suffered from housing deprivation. The
coefficients for smoking and excessive drinking
should be treated as a minimum estimate, since there
is only a limited amount of information on these
factors in the early sweeps. While it is important to
bear in mind the caveats regarding the robustness of
the index (see Chapter 5), the analysis indicates
strongly that housing deprivation was independently
associated with 'poor' health outcomes after
controlling for the other variables in the model.

Table 19: Stepwise Cox's regression results for the most significant variables that cause 'disability or severe' ill-health among cohort members in the NCDS

Variable	Odds ratio	95% confidence interval	Significance
HOUSING DEPRIVATION	1.08	1.06-1.11	0.000
SEX	1.11	1.06-1.16	0.000
CONGENITAL	1.95	1.68-2.25	0.000
DIVORCE	1.22	1.05-1.41	0.008
SMOKING	1.22	1.11-1.35	0.000
DRINKING	1.15	1.04-1.27	0.007

The Cox's regression model in Table 19 uses the
housing deprivation indices from the five sweeps.
In order to clarify the effects of multiple housing
deprivation on ill-health a second modelling
exercise was performed with the housing
deprivation indices dichotomised. For each sweep
each cohort member was allocated to a category as
either having 'no housing deprivation or a score of
one' or having 'two or more housing deprivations'.
Thus, multiple housing deprivation is defined for

each sweep as experiencing at least two housing deprivations. Each cohort member could have experienced multiple housing deprivation anywhere between zero and five times. As demonstrated in Chapter 5, Table 15, experiencing multiple deprivation in at least one sweep was quite common, while experiencing multiple deprivation in more than one sweep was relatively uncommon (fewer than one in five cohort members experienced multiple deprivation more than once).

Table 20 shows that the odds ratio for the increased risk of severe ill-health caused by multiple housing deprivation increased to 1.25 (1.16-1.34; 95% CI) after allowing for the effects of the other variables in the model. The results of this analysis are clear: multiple housing deprivation led to a 25% (on average) greater risk of disability or severe ill-health across the life-course of the cohort members in the NCDS. Thus, as one might expect in the light of the previous results indicating the strength of the associations between health and housing deprivation, when the longitudinal analysis focuses upon those who have experienced greater housing deprivation during childhood or early adulthood, the housing-related risk to health increases.

Table 20: Stepwise Cox's regression results for the most significant variables that cause 'disability or severe' ill-health among cohort members in the NCDS

Variable	Odds ratio	95% confidence interval	Significance
MULTIPLE HOUSING DEPRIVATION	1.25	1.16-1.34	0.000
SEX	1.11	1.06-1.16	0.000
CONGENITAL	1.94	1.68-2.24	0.000
DIVORCE	1.23	1.06-1.43	0.005
SMOKING	1.22	1.11-1.35	0.000
DRINKING	1.15	1.04-1.27	0.008

It is important to recognise that there is likely to be some error attached to this estimate, since many of the housing deprivation variables measured in the later sweeps of the NCDS were neither very reliable nor highly valid indicators of housing deprivation: they were more suited to measuring housing deprivation in the 1890s than the 1990s. A more appropriate index of housing deprivation would

yield much more accurate results: whether this would see the effect of housing deprivation strengthened or attenuated cannot be established a priori.

Interpretation

While our analysis points to the conclusion that housing conditions have a potentially significant impact upon the risk of ill-health, there are two competing interpretations of these results which could be offered. The first is the possibility that the relationships identified are a product of a health selection process, whereby as a result of experiencing poorer health, households find themselves in adverse housing circumstances. The second hypothesis is that households in poorer socio-economic circumstances – including housing circumstances – tend to have a more negative 'world-view' than other households and hence are more likely to report moderate or severe ill-health.

The housing-related health selection argument is an idea particularly associated with Smith (Smith, 1990). The argument is that two key processes are in operation. First, while a medical priority system operates in the allocation of social housing, bureaucratic discretion coupled with a shrinking social sector stock means that only those with medical needs who are also able to negotiate the system access social sector accommodation. Furthermore, even where access is gained to the social housing stock the fact that it was mostly higher quality stock that was sold under the Right to Buy process means that anyone living in the social sector has an increased probability of finding themselves in relatively poor housing conditions. Second, the competing demands upon the declining housing resources of the social sector mean that a sizeable proportion of those who have medical priority in principle must provide their own housing solutions in the private sector. In the private sector, ability to pay is the key determinant of access to quality accommodation and those with medical needs are likely to have restricted potential for earning income or labour market participation. Hence they will find themselves living at the lower end of the private market. These two processes in tandem will lead, it is argued, to those in lower health finding themselves in poorer housing conditions, but the poor housing conditions should more appropriately be seen as an effect rather than a cause of poor health.

While this account is clearly plausible, it is important to note that all health selection arguments are controversial and that, as we noted in Chapter 2, empirical work which has sought to test for health selection in the broader areas of social class or employment position – where such a mechanism is perhaps likely to be more immediate or direct – found little evidence for the operation of such effects. We are not aware of studies that examine in detail the possibility of an independent health selection effect that is the product of the operation of the housing market (see Smith and Mallinson, 1997b). At present, therefore, the health selection process in housing remains a plausible hypothesis which deserves to be investigated fully. However, with regard to the NCDS data, if health selection through housing were operating then it would most probably be acting through the health of the cohort member's parents rather than the cohort member himself/herself.

The hypothesis that households in poorer socio-economic circumstances tend to have a more negative 'world-view' than other households, and hence are more likely to report moderate or severe ill-health, needs to be addressed with three points. The argument assumes that the ill-health being considered is self-reported and it is this self-reporting which renders the information unreliable. In the case of the NCDS, the data from childhood relies upon medical examinations and, while the data in adulthood is self-reported, this analysis focuses upon medical conditions – such as, for example, kidney failure – which are not likely to be affected substantially by self-reporting bias. We do not consider that self-reporting bias is likely to be a significant source of error in this instance.

Even if the analysis relied upon self-reported health data, the argument for the impact of a 'negative world-view' held by disadvantaged households ignores the considerable epidemiological evidence that 'poor' and 'elderly' people tend to under-report their ill-health compared to 'younger' and 'richer' people. This is because both elderly and poor people are more likely to have experienced ill-health and therefore to have lower expectations of

good health than others. Furthermore, there is accumulating evidence that disproportionately more health resources go to 'richer' households than to 'poorer' households, given the health inequalities that exist. One of the controlling factors on the receipt of such services is demand: if poor people had a 'negative world-view' leading to reported ill-health then they would demand and receive more services. Yet, there is a range of evidence suggesting that better-off, middle-class people receive more health services relative to need than the poor (see Majeed et al, 1994; Worrall et al, 1997; Ben Shlomo and Chaturvedi, 1995; Chaturvedi and Ben Shlomo, 1995; Chaturvedi et al, 1997). Similar results have been reported for a range of other local services (see Bramley and Smart, 1993).

We therefore consider that the most appropriate interpretation of our results is that housing deprivation has a substantial impact upon the risk of ill-health. Considering these results in combination with the evidence on biomedical mechanisms from existing studies, briefly reviewed in Chapter 2, allows the construction of a fuller picture of the nature of the relationships involved. More evidence to corroborate the existing results and to isolate more precisely the mechanisms involved is always desirable, but existing evidence is now fairly extensive and points to the conclusion that the identified impact of housing deprivation upon risk of ill-health is indicative of a causal relationship.

Summary

After allowing for the effect of a range of genetic, behavioural, social and standard of living factors upon health, three housing-related variables emerged as important in increasing the odds of severe/moderate ill-health among cohort members at age 33. The factors, in order of importance, were: living in non-self-contained accommodation, past experience of homelessness and dissatisfaction with the area in which they were living.

When analysed longitudinally, genetic, social and behavioural factors emerge as significantly increasing a cohort member's likelihood of severe ill-health. Alongside these factors, level of housing deprivation also emerges as an independent source of increased likelihood of ill-health. When the analysis is repeated with the focus on whether cohort members suffered from multiple housing deprivation (two or more housing deprivations at a particular sweep), the effect of housing deprivation becomes stronger.

7

Implications

Exploring housing deprivation and health

This study is innovative in incorporating an index of housing deprivation, as the means of capturing adverse housing circumstances at different points in time, into an analysis of the factors influencing health. Many studies rely upon single or simple measures such as overcrowding or lack of amenities. Single measures are less desirable than a robust composite measure, especially when, as we demonstrate, some of the common single measures do not capture adequately the nature of deprivation. The study is also innovative in using a severity of ill-health index as the measure of health. The possibility of such an index has been discussed in the literature but this is the first study to operationalise one. By incorporating housing deprivation into an analysis which attempts to investigate the influence of the range of factors upon health, this study has demonstrated the gains that can be achieved from this approach.

It is important to recognise, however, that our analysis, like all secondary analysis, has been conducted within limits set by the available data. While the NCDS represents a particularly rich and wide-ranging data source, there are two important issues which need to be recognised when considering the implications of the analysis.

The first is that our attempt to create a housing deprivation index met with mixed success. The housing deprivation index used in this analysis drew on a range of NCDS housing variables encompassing physical characteristics, location, satisfaction, past homelessness and independent assessments of housing difficulties. The precise composition on the index varied between sweeps both because the sweeps gathered slightly different data and because the meaning and nature of deprivation changes over time and hence the most appropriate components for a deprivation index need to change if the index is to capture the phenomenon reliably.

The variables included in the indices were strongly associated with ill-health, but it became clear that while the housing-related questions in the NCDS had great relevance in the 1960s, their relevance declined rapidly such that for the later sweeps unreliable indices were being generated. While the NCDS data displays this feature, it is equally important to recognise that many of the other indices already in use have similar difficulties and that, in fact, the NCDS performs better than most. None the less, it would be desirable to explore this area further with a more reliable measure of housing deprivation.

The second issue that needs to be recognised relates to the link between housing deprivation and poverty. Perhaps the central concern for policy is whether housing deprivation has an effect upon health independent of the well-attested effects of low income. In order to examine this question fully it is desirable to have robust data on housing deprivation and income levels. Yet, the information on income which the NCDS offers cannot readily be employed in analysis. Our analysis relied on the alternative indicators of income levels – unemployment and the experience of financial difficulties – that were available. These indicators were included in the analysis and, while unemployment was found to be important in understanding ill-health at age 33, neither indicator was found to be important in explaining the probability of severe ill-health in the context of a longitudinal analysis. In contrast, housing deprivation was found to be an important influence in both cross-section and over time. Yet, the question as to whether an analysis that could include more accurate income data would lead to modified conclusions remains open.

Key messages to emerge from the research

In order to identify the key messages from this research it is important to consider the full range of the results presented. No single analysis or table can answer all the questions of interest.

Housing pathways

Tracing pathways of overcrowding and housing deprivation over time helps us to understand how the housing circumstances of a particular cohort have evolved and highlights the apparently diverse housing careers followed. Less than a quarter of cohort members never experienced any housing deprivation between birth and age 33, but long-term experience of multiple housing deprivation was relatively rare (only one in five cohort members experienced multiple deprivation during at least two sweeps).

When the focus is on overcrowding, evidence regarding its impact upon respiratory health and infectious disease is mixed. In childhood to age 11 it is associated with a heightened likelihood of experiencing infectious disease and in adulthood it is associated with increased likelihood of respiratory disease. While overcrowding in adulthood emerges strongly as a factor increasing the likelihood of respiratory disease, there was also evidence that experiencing overcrowding at birth and age 11 further increased the likelihood of suffering from respiratory disease. Broadening the analysis to consider the association between housing deprivation and ill-health more generally indicates that housing deprivation may play a role in increasing the likelihood of experiencing severe or moderate ill-health in adulthood and early childhood.

There are currently several competing interpretations of the role which housing or other socio-economic conditions may play in affecting health outcomes. Our analysis, when focused upon health and housing and without attempting to incorporate other types of risk, does not provide any strong support for the proposition that the accumulation of a 'chain' of housing deprivation risks throughout the life-course is a key factor in determining health in adulthood. That is not to say that housing deprivation may not interact with other health risks in a manner which results in a 'chain' of risks being formed which results in adverse health outcomes. In contrast, our analysis of housing deprivation, in isolation from other health risks, is more in accord with much of the existing literature which sees current conditions and, secondly, conditions in childhood as being the important influences on adult health. Yet, rather than assuming that this is the case the analysis examined housing deprivation in the intervening period and could not detect that it played a significant role in determining health in adulthood.

Housing in context

It is important to move beyond the examination of the relationship between housing and health in isolation and attempt to examine the influence of housing upon health in the context of the range of other factors which influence health in adulthood.

When housing circumstances in adulthood are analysed alongside other current influences upon health, three housing variables – whether the cohort member has been homeless, dissatisfied with the area they live in and living in non self-contained accommodation (rooms, caravans, etc) – emerge as significant explanatory variables even after controlling for other influences on health.

When housing deprivation is incorporated into a longitudinal analysis which seeks to address the range of factors – social, standard of living, genetic, behavioural – which can affect health, housing deprivation emerges as a very significant explanatory variable even after controlling for the other factors. Multiple housing deprivation led to a

25% (on average) greater risk of disability or severe ill-health across the life-course of the cohort members in the NCDS.

Housing and health

We would suggest that overall our analysis points to the conclusion that, once other factors have been controlled for, housing plays a significant role in health outcomes. The two exhibit a dose-response relationship: greater housing deprivation at a point in time will lead to greater probability of ill-health and a sustained experience of housing deprivation over time will increase the probability of ill-health. Equally important, housing history matters. Living in non-deprived housing conditions in adulthood is more likely to be associated with ill-health among those who have experienced housing deprivation earlier in life than among those who have not.

Implications of the research results for policy

The results of the longitudinal analysis strongly suggest that housing deprivation has a substantial effect upon the risk of ill-health. While it must be acknowledged that the NCDS data have limitations, the analysis that we have conducted is more comprehensive than existing analyses and this result can be considered reasonably well grounded.

Acting to improve the housing conditions of both adults and children would be of benefit. Addressing the housing conditions of children in particular would appear to deliver direct benefits in terms of improved current health and would also bring indirect benefits by reducing the likelihood of ill-health in later life. Further, our analysis reinforces existing findings regarding the deleterious effects of homelessness. Research has typically focused upon the association between current homelessness and current relatively poor health status. In contrast our focus is upon the impact of past homelessness upon current health. It indicates that those households who have experienced homelessness in the past had a considerably greater risk of current ill-health. While rehousing homeless households may attenuate the health injury associated with homelessness, it cannot remove it entirely.

Overall, it appears that for those living in circumstances of multiple housing deprivation, the risks of ill-health could be reduced significantly by action to tackle living conditions in deprived neighbourhoods, homelessness, and provide self-contained accommodation for all households. Based on the present analyses, the potential impact would appear to be of the same order of magnitude as tackling smoking or excessive alcohol consumption among members of the NCDS cohort.

These results have important implications for health policy. The thrust of current policy is very much in accord with the findings, recognising as it does the importance of socio-economic and environmental determinants of health status. Current policy debates place a welcome emphasis upon holistic approaches to health: in taking a more holistic view of the determinants of health, housing conditions need to be recognised as a significant influence.

It is important here to recall that our index of multiple housing deprivation goes beyond traditional concerns with the quality and amenities of a dwelling to incorporate key subjective factors such as satisfaction with dwelling or residential area. Thus tackling housing deprivation is not simply a question of raising housing standards, although addressing continuing problems of, for example, dampness and inadequate heating would clearly be welcome. Tackling deprivation is also about influencing the way in which residents perceive their accommodation and neighbourhood. Policy needs to address itself to the wider determinants of satisfaction.

Key current initiatives, such as Health Action Zones and Health Improvement Programmes, are founded on a recognition of the socio-economic determinants of health. And broader, regeneration-oriented initiatives, such as the New Deal for Communities, offer the opportunity both to reinforce such an holistic approach and to coordinate and target efforts on localities with particularly pressing needs. It is essential to ensure that the contribution that can be made by adequate housing to the health of adults and, particularly, children is never overlooked during implementation.

The emphasis in policy is increasingly upon the need for interdepartmental and joint working: our results suggest that for policy to have maximum impact upon health status housing issues and housing policies need to be an integral and important component of thinking and planning. Housing issues and housing organisations need to be given the necessary prominence in planning and resource allocation decisions at the local level if policy initiatives are to bring the greatest benefit to the health of local populations. Not only do health policy makers need to recognise the influence of housing on health status, but policy makers in housing and urban renewal need also to understand their potential contribution to achieving valuable health improvements and as a consequence be willing to play an active role in planning processes.

The duty to partnership which is being placed upon the organisations charged with implementing targets for health improvement provides a strong incentive for communication and working across disciplinary boundaries. Our research indicates that one of the most important boundaries that needs to be crossed is that between housing and health. 'Public health', as it has typically been conceived, could play an important role in ensuring that this boundary is effectively bridged.

In order that health policy at the local level can be fully effective not only do policy makers need to appreciate the important role of housing in influencing health status, but they also need to have available adequate data on the extent and distribution of housing deprivation locally. Such data need to be compiled on the basis of an appreciation of the nature of housing deprivation in the 1990s and need to be made available for consideration in all the relevant planning fora.

On a more specific policy issue, the emphasis placed upon the prevention of the most dramatic manifestation of homelessness – rough sleeping – by the Social Exclusion Unit (SEU, 1998) is addressing one key dimension of the health impact of housing. It is important to note that the homelessness referred to by the NCDS cohort members was not restricted to rough sleeping: those who had experienced homelessness may have experienced one or more types of insecure housing situation of which rough sleeping was only one. Hence, our analysis underlines the importance of recognising the health implications of a more broadly defined homelessness.

Contemporary policy at national level clearly recognises the type of issues we have identified. Housing is acknowledged to be one among a number of key influences upon health. Our analysis suggests that, from a longitudinal perspective, this is fully justified and that housing concerns should be an integral and explicit part of health policy. The key question is the extent to which implementation of the current agenda is able to deliver on its potential.

Methodological issues

The analysis reported above raises important methodological issues. The first relates to the desirability of a more reliable housing deprivation index. The analysis indicates strongly that there is a need to think about how we measure housing deprivation and about the data required to do so satisfactorily. Housing deprivation needs to be measured in relation to an appreciation of contemporary norms and consumption needs and patterns. A more reliable housing deprivation index requires the collection of data on housing circumstances and conditions that are appropriate and relevant to British society at the end of the 1990s. We believe that if such an analysis were undertaken then it would show a stronger effect than that which we identify, rather than demonstrating that housing deprivation does not make an important difference to health. Consequently it would represent a firmer base for action.

A second methodological point is that there would be a virtue in undertaking further development work on the NCDS in order to ensure that better quality income information were available. This would allow the analysis of the NCDS to advance further than we have been able to in this study.

A final methodological issue is that there is some evidence in the research literature that disease contracted in childhood can have long-lasting effects or can have effects that only become apparent after a considerable time lag. It may therefore be that the members of the NCDS cohort were not old enough in 1991 for the full import of certain types of infection or respiratory disease experienced in childhood as a result of adverse socio-economic conditions to become apparent. The proposed sweep to be conducted in 1999 provides an opportunity for any such longer-term consequences to begin to appear.

References

Abberley, P. (1996) 'Disabled by numbers', in R. Levitas and W. Guy (eds) *Interpreting official statistics*, London: Routledge, pp 166-79.

Acheson Report (1998) *Independent Inquiry into Inequalities in Health*, London: The Stationery Office.

Arblaster, L. and Hawtin, M. (1993) *Health, housing and social policy*, London: Socialist Health Association.

Ashmore, I. (1998) 'Asthma, housing and environmental health', *Environmental Health*, January, vol 106, pp 17-24.

Atkinson, A. (1985a) *How should we measure poverty? Some conceptual issues*, Discussion Paper 82, ESRC Programme on Taxation, Incentives and the Distribution of Income, London: London School of Economics.

Atkinson, A. (1985b) *On the measurement of poverty*, Discussion Paper 90, ESRC Programme on Taxation, Incentives and the Distribution of Income, London: London School of Economics.

Barker, D.J.P., Coggon, D., Osmond, C. and Wickham, C. (1990) 'Poor housing in childhood and high rates of stomach cancer in England and Wales', *British Journal of Cancer*, vol 61, pp 575-8.

Ben Shlomo, Y. and Chaturvedi, N. (1995) 'Assessing equity in access to health care provision in the UK: does where you live affect your chances of getting a CABG?', *Journal of Epidemiology and Community Health*, vol 49, pp 200-4.

Bines, W. (1997) 'The health of single homeless people', in R. Burrows, N. Pleace and D. Quilgars (eds) *Homelessness and social policy*, London: Routledge.

Blackburn C. (1990) *Poverty and health: Working with families*, Milton Keynes: Open University Press.

Blackman, T., Evason, E., Melaugh, M. and Woods, R. (1989) 'Housing and health: a case study of two areas in West Belfast', *Journal of Social Policy*, vol 18, no 1, pp 1-26.

Blane, D., Davey Smith, G., and Bartley, M. (1993) 'Social selection: what does it contribute to social class differentials in health?', *Sociology of Health and Illness*, vol 15, pp 1-15.

Blaxter, M. (1986) *Report on the longitudinal exploitation of the National Child Development Study: In areas of interest to the DHSS*, London: NCDS Working Paper No 7.

Blaxter, M. (1989) 'A comparison of measures of inequality in morbidity', in J. Fox (ed) *Health inequalities in european countries*, Aldershot: Gower.

Bone, M. and Meltzer, H. (1989) *The prevalence of disability among children*, OPCS surveys of disability in Great Britain, Report 3, London: HMSO.

Bor, W., Najman, J., Anderson, M., Morrison, J. and Williams, G. (1993) 'Socioeconomic disadvantage and child morbidity: an Australian longitudinal study', *Social Science & Medicine*, vol 36, pp 1053-61.

Bramley, G. and Smart, G. (1993) *Who benefits from local services?*, STICERD Working Paper 91, London: London School of Economics.

Breiman, L., Friedman, J.H., Olsten, R.A. and Stone, C.J. (1984) *Classification and regression trees*, Belmont, CA: Wadsworth.

Brittan, N., Davies, J.M.C. and Colley, J.R.T. (1987) 'Early respiratory experience and subsequent cough and peak expiratory flow rate in 36 year old men and women', *BMJ*, vol 294, pp 1317-20.

Brown, G.W. and Harris, T. (1978) *Social origins of depression: A study of psychiatric disorders in women*, London: Tavistock.

Burr, M., Mullins, J., Merrett, T. and Stott, N. (1988) 'Indoor moulds and asthma', *Journal of the Royal Society of Health*, vol 108, pp 99-102.

Chadwick, E. (1842) *Report on the sanitary conditions of the labouring population of Great Britain*, London: HMSO.

Chapman, M. (1993) 'Cockroach allergens: a common cause of asthma in North American cities', *Insights in Allergy*, vol 8, pp 1-8.

Chaturvedi, N. and Ben Shlomo, Y. (1995) 'From surgery to surgeon: does deprivation influence access to care?', *British Journal of General Practice*, vol 45, pp 127-31.

Chaturvedi, N., Rai, J. and Ben Shlomo, Y. (1997) 'Lay diagnosis and health care seeking behaviour for chest pain in South Asians and Europeans', *Lancet*, vol 350, pp 1578-83.

Coggon, D., Barker, D.J.P., Inskip, H. and Wield, G. (1993) 'Housing in early life and later mortality', *Journal of Epidemiology and Community Health*, vol 47, pp 345-8.

Collins, J. (1993) 'Cold and heat related illnesses in the indoor environment', in R. Burridge and D. Ormandy (eds) *Unhealthy housing, research remedies and reform*, London: E & FN Spon, pp 117-37.

Collins, K. (1986) 'Low indoor temperatures and morbidity in the elderly', *Age and Ageing*, vol 15, pp 212-20.

Conway, J. (1988) (ed) *Prescription for poor health. The crisis for homeless families*, London: London Food Commission, Maternity Alliance, SHAC, Shelter.

Conway, J. (1993) 'Ill-health and homelessness', in R. Burridge and D. Ormandy (eds) *Unhealthy housing, research remedies and reform*, London: E & FN Spon, pp 283-300.

Cook, D. and Strachen, D. (1997) 'Parental smoking and prevalence of respiratory symptoms and asthma in school age children', *Thorax*, vol 52, pp 1081-94.

Cronbach, L. (1951) 'Coefficient alpha and the internal structure of tests', *Psychometrica*, vol 16, pp 297-334.

Cronbach, L. (1976) *Research in classrooms and schools: Foundations of questions, design and analysis*, Stanford, CA: Stanford University Evaluation Consortium.

Cronbach, L. et al (1971) *The dependability of behavioural measurement*, New York, NY: Wiley.

Dales, R.E., Zwanenburg, H., Bumett, R. and Franklin, C.A. (1991) 'Respiratory health effects of home dampness and moulds among Canadian children', *American Journal of Epidemiology*, vol 134, pp 196-203.

Davey-Smith, G. and Phillips, A. (1992) 'Confounding in epidemiological studies: why "independent" effects may not be all they seem', *BMJ*, vol 305, pp 757-9.

Davey Smith, G., Hart, C., Blan, D., Gillis, C. and Hawthorne, V., (1997) 'Lifetime socioeconomic position and mortality: prospective observational study', *BMJ*, vol 314, pp 547-52.

Dekker, C., Dales, R., Bartlett, S., Brunekreef, B. and Zwanenburg, H. (1991) 'Childhood asthma and the indoor environment', *Chest*, vol 100, pp 922-6.

DoH (Department of Health) (1998) *Our Healthier Nation: A contract for health*, Cm 3852, London: The Stationery Office.

Donaldson, K.J. and Donaldson, L.J. (1983) *Essential community medicine*, Lancaster: MTP Press.

EEC (1985) *On specific community action to combat poverty* (Council Decision of 19 December 1984), 85/8/EEC, Office Journal of the EEC, 2/24.

EEC (1991) *Final report of the second European poverty programme 1985-1989*, Luxembourg: Office for the Official Publications of the European Communities.

Fanning, D. (1967) 'Families in flats', *BMJ*, pp 382-6.

Fogelman, K. (1976) *Britain's sixteen year olds*, London: National Children's Bureau.

Fox, J., Goldblatt, P. and Jones, D. (1985) 'Social-class mortality differentials: artefact, selection or life circumstances', *Journal of Epidemiology and Community Health*, vol 39, pp 1-8.

Freeman, H. (1993) 'Mental health and high-rise housing', in R. Burridge and D. Ormandy (eds) *Unhealthy housing, research remedies and reform*, London: E & FN Spon.

Gabe, J. and Williams, P. (1993) 'Women, crowding and mental health', in R. Burridge and D. Ormandy (eds) *Unhealthy housing, research remedies and reform*, London: E & FN Spon, pp 191-208.

Ghodsian, M. and Fogelman, K. (1988) *A longitudinal study of housing circumstances in childhood and early adulthood*, London: NCDS User Support Group Working Paper 29.

Gordon, D. (1995) 'Census based deprivation indices: their weighting and validation', *Journal of Epidemiology and Community Health*, vol 49 (Suppl 2), pp S39-S44.

Gordon, D. and Pantazis, C. (eds) (1997) *Breadline Britain in the 1990s*, Aldershot: Avebury.

Harris, A.I. (1971) *Handicapped and impaired in Great Britain*, London: HMSO.

Harvey, D. and Kovar, I. (1985) *A child health textbook for the DCH*, London: Churchill Livingstone.

Hopton, J. and Hunt, S. (1996) 'The health effects of improvements to housing: a longitudinal study', *Housing Studies*, vol 11, no 2, pp 271-86.

Hunt, S.M. (1990) 'Emotional distress and bad housing', *Health and Hygiene*, vol 11, pp 72-9.

Hunt, S.M. (1997) 'Housing-related disorders', in J. Charlton and M. Murphy (eds) *The health of adult Britain 1841-1994*, vol 1, Decennial Supplement No 12, London: The Stationery Office.

Hyndman, S. (1990) 'Housing dampness and health amongst British Bengalis in East London', *Social Science & Medicine*, vol 30, no 1, pp 131-41.

Ineichen, B. (1993) *Homes and health*, London: E & FN Spon.

Ineichen, B. and Hooper, D. (1974) 'Wives' mental health and children's behaviour problems in contrasting residential areas', *Social Science and Medicine*, vol 8, pp 369-74.

Kuh, D. and Ben-Shlomo, Y. (eds) (1997) *A life-course approach to chronic disease epidemiology*, Oxford: Oxford Medical Publications.

Kuh, D. and Wadsworth, M. (1989) 'Parental height, childhood environment and subsequent adult height in a national birth cohort', *International Journal of Epidemiology*, vol 18, pp 663-7.

Kurden, F. (1970) 'Some principles of interest measurement', *Educational Psychology*, vol 30, pp 205-26.

Leather, P., Mackintosh, S. and Rolfe, S. (1994) *Papering over the cracks: Housing conditions and the nation's health*, London: National Housing Forum.

Lee, P., Murie, A. and Gordon, D. (1995) *Area measures of deprivation: A study of current methods and best practices in the identification of poor areas in Great Britain*, Birmingham: University of Birmingham.

Lewis, G. and Ulph, D. (1988) 'Poverty, inequality and welfare', *Economic Journal*, vol 98 (Conference), pp 117-31.

Lowry, S. (1991) *Housing and Health*, London: British Medical Journal.

Mack, J. and Lansley, S. (1985) *Poor Britain*, London: Allen and Unwin.

Majeed, A., Chaturvedi, N., Reading, R. and Ben Shlomo, Y. (1994) 'Monitoring and promoting equity in primary and acute care', *BMJ*, vol 308, p 1426.

Mann, S.L., Wadsworth, M.E.J. and Colley, J.R.T. (1992) 'Accumulation of factors in influencing respiratory illness in members of a national birth cohort and their offspring', *Journal of Epidemiology and Community Health*, vol 46, pp 286-90.

Martin, J. and White, A. (1988) *Report 2: The financial circumstances of disabled adults in private households*, London: HMSO.

Martin, J., Meltzer, H. and Elliot, D. (1988) *Report 1: The prevalence of disability amongst adults*, London: HMSO.

Martin, J., White, A. and Meltzer, H. (1989) *Report 4: Disabled adults: Services, transport and employment*, London: HMSO.

Martyn, C. (1991) 'Childhood infection and adult disease', *Ciba Foundation Symposia*, vol 156, pp 93-108.

Mendall, M.A., Goggin, P.M., Molineaux, N., Levy, J., Toosy, T., Strachan, D. and Northfield, T.C. (1992) 'Childhood living conditions and *Helicobacter pylori* seropositivity in adult life', *Lancet*, vol 339, pp 896-7.

Meltzer, H., Smyth, M. and Robus, N. (1989) *Report 6: Disabled children: Services, transport and education*, London: HMSO.

Miller, J.D. (1992) 'Fungi as contaminants in indoor air', *Atmospheric Environment Part A*, vol 26, pp 2163-72.

Montgomery, S., Bartley, M. and Wilkinson, R. (1996) *The association of slow growth in childhood with family conflict*, London: NCDS User Support Group Working Paper No 48.

Mood, E. (1993) 'Fundamentals of healthful housing: their application in the 21st century', in R. Burridge and D. Ormandy (eds) *Unhealthy housing: research, remedies and reform*, London: E & FN Spon, pp 304-34.

Murie, A. (1983) *Housing inequality and deprivation*, London: Heinemann.

Murray, R. (1974) 'The influence of crowding on children's behaviour', in D. Canter and T. Lee (eds) *Psychology and the built environment*, London: Architectural Press.

Nunnally, J. (1981) *Psychometric theory*, New Delhi: Tate-Mcgraw-Hill.

Packer, C., Stewart-Brown, S. and Fowle, S. (1994) 'Damp housing and adult health: results from a life-style study in Worcester, England', *Journal of Epidemiology and Community Health*, vol 48, pp 555-9.

Payne, S. (1991) *Women, health and poverty: An introduction*, Hemel Hempstead: Harvester Wheatsheaf.

Payne, S. (1997) 'Poverty and mental health', in D. Gordon and C. Pantazis (eds) *Breadline Britain in the 1990s*, Aldershot: Avebury.

Piachaud, D. (1987) 'Problems in the definition and measurement of poverty', *Journal of Social Policy*, vol 16, no 2, pp 147-64.

Platt, S., Martin, C. and Hunt, S. (1989) 'Damp housing, mould growth and symptomatic health state', *BMJ*, vol 298, pp 1673-8.

Platt-Mills, T. and Chapman, M. (1987) 'Dust mite: immunology, allergic disease and environmental control', *Journal of Allergy and Clinical Immunology*, vol 80, pp 755-75.

Power, C. (1991) 'Social and economic background and class inequalities in health among young adults', *Social Science and Medicine*, vol 32, no 4, pp 411-17.

Power, C., Fox, A. J., Manor, O. and Fogelman, K. (1988) The role of health selection in explaining class differences in health in the NCDS'. NCDS Working Paper No 28. London: Social Statistics Research Unit, City University.

Power, C. and Hertzman, C. (1997) 'Social and biological pathways linking early life and adult disease', in M. Marmot and M. Wadsworth (eds) 'Fetal and early childhood environment: Long-term health implications', *British Medical Bulletin*, vol 53, no 1, pp 210-23.

Power, C., Hertzman, C., Matthews, S. and Manor, O. (1997) 'Social differences in health: life-cycle effects between ages 23 and 33 in the 1958 British birth cohort', *American Journal of Public Health*, vol 87, no 9, pp 1499-503.

Power, C., Manor, O. and Fox, J. (1991) *Health and class: The early years*, London: Chapman and Hall.

Power, C., Matthews, S. and Manor, O. (1996) 'Inequalities in self rated health in the 1958 birth cohort: lifetime social circumstances or social mobility?', *BMJ*, vol 313, pp 449-53.

Power. C. and Matthews, S. (1997) 'Origins of health inequalities in a national population sample', *Lancet*, vol 350, pp 1584-9.

Power, C. and Peckham, C. (1988) *Childhood morbidity and adult ill-health*, London: NCDS Working Paper No 32.

Power, C. and Peckham, C. (1990) 'Childhood morbidity and adult ill-health', *Journal of Epidemiology and Community Health*, vol 44, pp 69-74.

Reading, R. (1997) 'Social disadvantage and infection in childhood', *Sociology of health and illness*, vol 19, pp 395-414.

Robinson, D. (1998) 'Health selection in the housing system: access to council housing for homeless people with health problems', *Housing Studies*, vol 13, no 1, pp 23-41.

Rona, R.J. and Chinn, S. (1993) 'Lung-function, respiratory illness and passive smoking in British primary-school children', *Thorax*, vol 48, pp 21-5.

Rutter, M. (1974) 'Attainment and adjustment in two geographical areas: some factors accounting for area differences', *British Journal of Psychiatry*, vol 125, pp 520-33.

SEU (Social Exclusion Unit) (1998) *Rough sleeping*, Cm 4008, London: The Stationery Office.

Shanks, N. and Smith, S.J. (1992) 'Public policy and the health of homeless people', *Policy & Politics*, vol 20, no 1, pp 35-46.

Shepherd, P. (1995) *The National Child Development Study: An introduction, its origins and the methods of data collection*, NCDS User Support Group Working Paper No 1, London: City University.

Smith, S.J. (1989) *Housing and health: A review and research agenda*, Discussion Paper No 27, Glasgow: Centre for Housing Research, Glasgow University.

Smith, S.J. (1990) 'Health status and the housing system', *Social Science and Medicine*, vol 31, pp 753-62.

Smith, S.J. and Mallinson, S. (1997a) 'The problem with social housing: discretion, accountability and the welfare ideal', *Policy & Politics*, vol 24, pp 339-57.

Smith, S.J. and Mallinson, S. (1997b) 'Housing for health in a post-welfare state', *Housing Studies*, vol 12, no 2, pp 173-200.

Smyth, M. and Robus, N. (1989) *Report 5: The financial circumstances of disabled children living in private households*, London: HMSO.

Southgate, I., Lockie, C., Heard, S. and Wood, M. (1997) *Infection*, Oxford: Oxford Medical Publications.

Spearman, C. (1904) 'General intelligence objectively determined and measured', *American Journal of Psychology*, vol 15, pp 201-93.

Spengler, J., Neas, L., Nakai, S., Dockery, D., Speizer, F., Ware, J. and Raizenne, M. (1994) 'Respiratory symptoms and housing characteristics', *Indoor Air*, vol 4, pp 72-82.

Sporik, R., Chapman, M. and Platt-Mills, T. (1992) 'House dust mite exposure as a cause of asthma', *Clinical Experimental Allergy*, vol 22, pp 897-906.

Stanley, D. (1971) 'Reliability', in R. Thorndike (ed) *Educational measurement*, Washington, DC: American Council on Education.

Stewart, W. (1970) *Children in flats: A family study*, London: NSPCC.

Strachan, D. and Elton, P. (1986) 'The relationship between respiratory morbidity in children and the home environment', *Family Practice*, vol 3, pp 137-42.

Strachan, D. and Sanders, C. (1989) 'Damp housing and childhood asthma: respiratory effects of indoor air temperature and relative humidity', *Journal of Epidemiology and Community Health*, vol 43, pp 7-14.

Sutherland, A. and Chesson, R. (1994) 'Open to question', *Health Service Journal*, 21 April, vol 104.

Thunhurst, C. (1993) 'Using published data to assess health risks', in R. Burridge and D. Ormandy (eds) *Unhealthy housing: Research, remedies and reform*, London: E & FN Spon.

Tobin, R., Baranowski, E., Gilman, A. et al (1987) 'The significance of fungi in indoor air', *Canadian Journal of Public Health*, vol 78 (suppl), pp 1-14.

Townsend, P. (1979) *Poverty in the United Kingdom*, Harmondsworth: Penguin.

Townsend, P. (1987) 'Deprivation', *Journal of Social Policy*, vol 16, no 2, pp 125-46.

Townsend, P. (1993) *The international analysis of poverty*, Milton Keynes: Harvester Wheatsheaf.

Townsend, P. and Gordon, D. (1993) *What is enough? New evidence on poverty in Greater London allowing the definition of a minimum benefit*, Memorandum of Evidence to the House of Commons Social Services Select Committee on Minimum Income, vol 579, pp 45-73.

Universities of Sussex and Westminster (1996) *The real cost of poor homes*, London: Royal Institution of Chartered Surveyors.

Verhoeff, A., Van Strien, R., Van Wijnen, J. and Brunekreef, B. (1995) 'Damp housing and childhood respiratory symptoms: the role of sensitization to dust mites and molds', *American Journal of Epidemiology*, vol 141, pp 103-10.

Weitzman, M., Gortmaker, S., Walker, D. and Sobol, A. (1990) 'Maternal smoking and childhood asthma', *Pediatrics*, vol 85, pp 505-11.

West, P. (1988) 'Inequalities? Social class differentials in health in British youth', *Social Science and Medicine*, vol 27, pp 291-6.

Williamson, I., Martin, C., McGill, G., Monie, R. and Fennerty, A. (1997) 'Damp housing and asthma: a case control study', *Thorax*, vol 52, pp 229-34.

Worrall, A., Rea, J. and Ben Shlomo, Y. (1997) 'Counting the cost of social disadvantage in primary care: retrospective analysis of patient data', *BMJ*, vol 314, pp 38-42.

Wyke, S., Hewison, J., Hey, E. and Russell, I. (1991) 'Respiratory illness in children: do deprived children have worse coughs?', *Acta Paediatrica Scandinavica*, vol 80, pp 704-11.

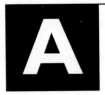

Appendix A: Details of the items included in each scale of each 'health measure'

	Sweep 1 (1965)	Sweep 2 (1969)	Sweep 3 (1974)	Sweep 4 (1981)	Sweep 5 (1991)
'Disabled/ severe health problem'	In special education	In special education	In special education	Is registered disabled	Is registered disabled
	and/or	*and/or*	*and/or*	*and/or*	*and/or*
	Mother reports physical handicap/ disability		Mother reports physical handicap/ disability	Declares *limiting* long-standing illness, disability or infirmity	Declares *limiting* long-standing illness, disability or infirmity
	and/or	*and/or*	*and/or*	*and/or*	*and/or*
		Has had an epileptic fit during the past year	Has had an epileptic fit during the past year	Has had an epileptic fit during the past year	Has had an epileptic fit during the past year
	and/or	*and/or*	*and/or*	*and/or*	*and/or*
	Moderate or severe handicap noted at medical examination	Doctor reports physical handicap/ disability	Moderate or severe handicap noted at medical examination	Is out of the workforce permanently because sick or disabled	Is out of the workforce permanently because sick or disabled
	and/or	*and/or*	*and/or*	*and/or*	*and/or*
	Does not have normal bowel control	Does not have normal bowel control/ or is wet day or night	Does not have normal bowel control/ or is wet day or night	Is in receipt of invalidity benefit/attendance allowance/ mobility allowance	Is in receipt of invalidity benefit/attendance allowance/ mobility allowance
				and/or	
				Currently works in sheltered workshop	

Appendix A continued

Sweep 1 (1965)	Sweep 2 (1969)	Sweep 3 (1974)	Sweep 4 (1981)	Sweep 5 (1991)
'Moderate health problem' (if not already included in above group)	Has chronic physical, medical or sensory conditions, asthma or psychosocial problems	Has chronic physical, medical or sensory conditions, asthma or psychosocial problems	Has chronic physical, medical or sensory conditions, asthma or psychosocial problems	Declares *non-limiting* long-standing illness, disability or infirmity	Declares *non-limiting* long-standing illness, disability or infirmity
	and/or	*and/or*	*and/or*	*and/or*	*and/or*
	Slight handicap noted at medical examination	Medical examination suggests hearing or visual problems will affect schooling	Slight handicap noted at medical examination	Receives any *regular* medical supervision	Receives any *regular* medical supervision
		and/or	*and/or*	*and/or*	*and/or*
		More than one month off school in past year for ill-health	More than one month off school in past year for ill-health	Is under medical supervision for epilepsy or asthma	Is under medical supervision for epilepsy or asthma, heart trouble, high blood pressure or cancer
				and/or	*and/or*
				Has had two or more hospital admissions in past year	Has had two or more hospital admissions in past year
				and/or	and/or
				Seen specialist for psychiatric problems in past year	Seen specialist for psychiatric problems since age 23 and current symptoms
				and/or	*and/or*
				Description of own health 'poor'	Description of own health 'poor'

Appendix A continued

	Sweep 1 (1965)	Sweep 2 (1969)	Sweep 3 (1974)	Sweep 4 (1981)	Sweep 5 (1991)
'Some health problems' (if not already included in above groups)	Has allergic or psychosomatic conditions	Has allergic or psychosomatic conditions	Has allergic or psychosomatic conditions	Has cough/ phlegm in winter	Has cough/ phlegm in winter
	and/or	*and/or*	*and/or*	*and/or*	*and/or*
	Some (non-handicapping medical condition noted at medical examination	Some (non-handicapping medical condition noted at medical examination	Some (non-handicapping medical condition noted at medical examination	Last consulted GP less than 6 months ago about own health	Last consulted GP/specialist within past year about named condition
		and/or	*and/or*	*and/or*	*and/or*
		Has been admitted to hospital 3 times or more since age 7	Has been admitted to hospital in past year	Has been admitted to hospital in past year	Has been admitted to hospital in past year
			and/or		*and/or*
			Has attended out patient clinic in past year		Declares health in past year to be 'not so good'
		and/or	*and/or*		*and/or*
		Recent fractured bone	Recent fractured bone		Has had work -absence because of back pain
'No health problems'	All other cohort members in survey	All other cohort members in survey	All other cohort members in survey	All other cohort members in survey	All other cohort members in survey

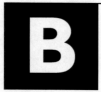

Appendix B: Analytical methods

Chi-squared automatic interaction detector methodology

The chi-squared automatic interaction detector (CHAID) methodology is based on an algorithm developed by Kass in 1980 and has only recently become available as an add-in to the SPSS statistical package. It belongs to a family of techniques known as classification trees, which includes Automatic Interaction Detector (AID) and Classification and Regression Trees (CART) techniques. These techniques can be used to perform discriminant analysis on categorical data.

The relative newness of these techniques means that little is known about them. However, CHAID has the advantage that it can produce intuitive, easy to understand, classification rules. It can also identify sub-groupings within the data that would be impossible to detect with conventional techniques.

In 1988, the US Committee on Applied and Theoretical Statistics' expert panel on Discriminant and Cluster Analysis considered that the status of classification trees was best summarised by the main developers (Breiman et al, 1984):

Binary trees give an interesting and often illuminating way of looking at data in classification or regression problems. They should not be used to the exclusion of other methods. We do not claim they are always better. They do add a flexible nonparametric tool to the data analyst's arsenal.

Logistic regression

In order to examine component validity ordinal logistic regression was used with the health index (coded 1 to 4, that is, no health problems to severe/disabled) as a response variable, that is, the health index was not dichotomise but was treated as an ordinal variable.

Nominal logistic regression also allowed the use of all four categories of the health index but they were treated as a categorical variable, that is, not as an ordinal scale going from 'best' health to 'worst' health. In order to run the binary logistic models the health index had to be dichotomised into 'severe/moderate ill-health' and 'minor/no ill-health'.

The summary results listed in the tables in Appendix C are from ordinary binary logistic regression, ordinal logistic regression and nominal logistic regression.

The reasons for using ordinal and nominal models are as follows;

- Ordinal logistic regression allows the health index to be treated as an ordinal scale and also allows three different distributional models to be fitted:

  Logistic   –   The model has a logistic distribution

  Probit   –   The model has a normal distribution

  Gompit   –   The model has a Gompertz (log-log) distribution

If significant results can be demonstrated using different assumptions about the nature of the data then this provides support for the view that the results are not the product of the particular estimation technique.

- Nominal logistic regression allows all four categories of the health index to be used but without the assumption of an ordinal scale. Therefore, for example, it allows the test to determine if the fourth category 'disabled/severe' is actually worse than the third category 'moderate ill-health'. It might be that 'disabled' people are not unhealthy, that is, they might be 'disabled' but not 'sick'.

The nominal logistic regression with the health index as the dependent variable yields three sets of results, for example, the effect of each housing deprivation variable on 'No health problem' versus 'Minor problems', 'No health problem' versus 'Moderate problems' and 'No health problem' versus 'Disabled/severe problems'.

The reliability of measurement

The theory of measurement error has been developed mainly by psychologists and educationalists and its origins can be traced to the work of Spearman (1904). The most widely used model is the Domain-Sampling Model, although many of the key equations can be derived from other models based on different assumptions (see Nunnally, 1981, Chapters 5-9, for detailed discussion). The Domain-Sampling Model assumes that there is an infinite number of questions (or, at least, a large number of questions) that could be asked about housing deprivation. If you had an infinite amount of time, patience and research grant, you could ask every person/household all of these questions and then you would know everything about their level of housing deprivation, that is, you would know their 'true' housing deprivation score. The nine questions used in the 1965 sweep of the NCDS when the children were aged 7 can be considered to be a subset of this larger group (domain) of all possible questions about housing deprivation (Gordon and Pantazis, 1997).

Some questions will obviously be better at measuring deprivation than others; however, all of the questions that measure deprivation will have some common core. If they do not, they are not measuring deprivation by definition. Therefore, all the questions that measure deprivation should be intercorrelated such that the sum (or average) of all the correlations of one question, with all the others, will be the same for all questions (Nunnally, 1981). If this assumption is correct, then by measuring the average intercorrelation between the answers to the set of deprivation questions, it is possible to calculate both:

- an estimate of the correlation between the set of questions and the 'true' scores that would be obtained if the infinite set of all possible deprivation questions had been asked; and

- the average correlation between the set of questions asked (the deprivation index) and all other possible sets of deprivation questions (deprivation indices) of equal length (equal number of questions).

Both these correlations can be derived from Cronbach's coefficient alpha which, when transformed for use with dichotomous questions, is known as KR-20, short for Kurder-Richardson Formula 20 (Cronbach, 1951, 1976; Cronbach et al, 1971; Kurder, 1970).

The coefficient alpha is 0.688 for the nine questions in sweep 1 of the NCDS, for example. This is the average correlation between these nine questions and all the other possible sets of nine questions that could be used to measure housing deprivation. The estimated correlation between these nine NCDS housing deprivation questions and the 'true' scores, from the infinite possible number of housing deprivation questions, is the square root of coefficient alpha, that is, 0.8294.

Nunnally (1981) has argued that:

> *... in the early stages of research ... one saves time and energy by working with instruments that have modest reliability, for which purpose reliabilities of 0.70 or higher will suffice ... for basic research, it can be argued that increasing reliabilities much beyond 0.80 is often wasteful of time and funds, at that level correlations are attenuated very little by measurement error.*

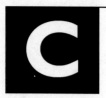

Appendix C: Detailed results

The tables in each of the following sections are ordered by approximate level of significance of the ordinal logistic regression results.

Housing deprivation in 1965

Table 1: Logistic regression results for housing difficulties recorded by the health visitor at age 7

Model	Odds/Z score	95% confidence interval	Significance
Binary logistic	1.46	1.28-1.67	0.000
Ordinal – logistic	1.41	1.24-1.59	0.000
Ordinal – probit	5.35		0.000
Ordinal – gompit	4.82		0.000
Nominal – none vs minor	1.03	0.86-1.24	0.739
Nominal – none vs moderate	1.45	1.23-1.72	0.000
Nominal – none vs severe	1.74	1.29-2.33	0.000

Table 2: Logistic regression results for not having sole access to hot water at age 7

Model	Odds/Z score	95% confidence interval	Significance
Binary logistic	1.32	1.17-1.50	0.000
Ordinal – logistic	1.33	1.19-1.49	0.000
Ordinal – probit	5.13		0.000
Ordinal – gompit	4.60		0.000
Nominal – none vs minor	1.13	0.96-1.34	0.149
Nominal – none vs moderate	1.35	1.15-1.58	0.000
Nominal – none vs severe	1.88	1.43-2.45	0.000

Table 3: Logistic regression results for overcrowding at age 7

Model	Odds/Z score	95% confidence interval	Significance
Binary logistic	1.22	1.14-1.32	0.000
Ordinal – logistic	1.19	1.11-1.27	0.000
Ordinal – probit	5.50 (Z-score)		0.000
Ordinal – gompit	3.69 (Z-score)		0.000
Nominal – none vs minor	0.94	0.86-1.04	0.229
Nominal – none vs moderate	1.13	1.04-1.24	0.006
Nominal – none vs severe	1.68	1.41-1.99	0.000

Table 4: Logistic regression results for lacking or sharing an indoor toilet at age 7

Model	Odds/Z score	95% confidence interval	Significance
Binary logistic	1.20	1.10 – 1.32	0.000
Ordinal – logistic	1.19	1.10 – 1.30	0.000
Ordinal – probit	4.30		0.000
Ordinal- gompit	3.44		0.001
Nominal – none vs minor	1.02	0.90 – 1.15	0.728
Nominal – none vs moderate	1.17	1.05 – 1.32	0.006
Nominal – none vs severe	1.55	1.26 – 1.91	0.000

Table 5: Logistic regression results for not having sole access to a bath at age 7

Model	Odds/Z score	95% confidence interval	Significance
Binary logistic	1.18	1.06-1.31	0.002
Ordinal – logistic	1.18	1.07-1.30	0.001
Ordinal – probit	3.63		0.000
Ordinal – gompit	2.84		0.005
Nominal – none vs minor	1.03	0.90-1.19	0.658
Nominal – none vs moderate	1.15	1.01-1.31	0.039
Nominal – none vs severe	1.59	1.26-2.01	0.000

Table 6: Logistic regression results for children living in non-self-contained accommodation at age 7

Model	Odds/Z score	95% confidence interval	Significance
Binary logistic	1.12	0.93-1.35	0.226
Ordinal – logistic	1.14	0.97-1.36	0.117
Ordinal – probit	1.74		0.082
Ordinal – gompit	1.36		0.173
Nominal – none vs minor	1.06	0.83-1.36	0.627
Nominal – none vs moderate	1.11	0.88-1.40	0.396
Nominal – none vs severe	1.55	1.04-2.32	0.032

Table 7: Logistic regression results for not having sole access to a garden or yard at age 7

Model	Odds/Z score	95% confidence interval	Significance
Binary logistic	1.10	0.97-1.25	0.125
Ordinal – logistic	1.07	0.96-1.20	0.224
Ordinal – probit	1.26		0.206
Ordinal – gompit	0.72		0.472
Nominal – none vs minor	0.93	0.79-1.10	0.420
Nominal – none vs moderate	1.05	0.90-1.22	0.552
Nominal – none vs severe	1.21	0.91-1.62	0.198

Table 8: Logistic regression results for not having sole access to a cooker at age 7

Model	Odds/Z score	95% confidence interval	Significance
Binary logistic	1.10	0.75-1.62	0.626
Ordinal – logistic	0.96	0.68-1.37	0.832
Ordinal – probit	0.13		0.895
Ordinal – gompit	-1.10		0.271
Nominal – none vs minor	0.51	0.30-0.87	0.013
Nominal – none vs moderate	0.70	0.44-1.11	0.134
Nominal – none vs severe	1.75	0.89-3.43	0.105

Table 9: Logistic regression results for children living in flats at age 7

Model	Odds/Z score	95% confidence interval	Significance
Binary logistic	1.00	0.88-1.15	0.970
Ordinal – logistic	0.97	0.86-1.10	0.640
Ordinal – probit	-0.45		0.656
Ordinal – gompit	-0.79		0.431
Nominal – none vs minor	0.89	0.75-1.06	0.200
Nominal – none vs moderate	0.94	0.80-1.11	0.481
Nominal – none vs severe	0.99	0.71-1.36	0.929

Housing deprivation in 1969

Table 10: Logistic regression results for mother unsatisfied or very unsatisfied with accommodation at age 11

Model	Odds/Z score	95% confidence interval	Significance
Binary logistic	1.51	1.36-1.67	0.000
Ordinal – logistic	1.59	1.45-1.74	0.000
Ordinal – probit	10.02		0.000
Ordinal – gompit	10.46		0.000
Nominal – none vs minor	1.51	1.32-1.74	0.000
Nominal – none vs moderate	1.67	1.45-1.92	0.000
Nominal – none vs severe	2.11	1.81-2.46	0.000

Table 11: Logistic regression results for mother unsatisfied with the location of the accommodation at age 11

Model	Odds/Z score	95% confidence interval	Significance
Binary logistic	1.49	1.28-1.74	0.000
Ordinal – logistic	1.64	1.42-1.88	0.000
Ordinal – probit	7.09		0.000
Ordinal – gompit	6.91		0.000
Nominal – none vs minor	1.48	1.20-1.83	0.000
Nominal – none vs moderate	1.45	1.16-1.81	0.000
Nominal – none vs severe	2.36	1.89-2.96	0.000

Table 12: Logistic regression results for children living in flats at age 11

Model	Odds/Z score	95% confidence interval	Significance
Binary logistic	1.42	1.26-1.60	0.000
Ordinal – logistic	1.44	1.29-1.60	0.000
Ordinal – probit	6.59		0.000
Ordinal – gompit	7.46		0.000
Nominal – none vs minor	1.43	1.23-1.68	0.000
Nominal – none vs moderate	1.70	1.45-1.99	0.000
Nominal – none vs severe	1.64	1.37-1.97	0.000

Table 13: Logistic regression results for child living in accommodation with a front door on or above the third floor of the building at age 11

Model	Odds/Z score	95% confidence interval	Significance
Binary logistic	1.38	1.07-1.78	0.000
Ordinal – logistic	1.41	1.12-1.77	0.003
Ordinal – probit	2.88		0.004
Ordinal – gompit	3.40		0.001
Nominal – none vs minor	1.49	1.06-2.09	0.023
Nominal – none vs moderate	1.71	1.21-2.42	0.002
Nominal – none vs severe	1.59	1.07-2.38	0.023

Table 14: Logistic regression results for mother unsatisfied with the comfort, manageability, 'ease of running' or modern amenities of the accommodation at age 11

Model	Odds/Z score	95% confidence interval	Significance
Binary logistic	1.34	1.19-1.51	0.000
Ordinal – logistic	1.40	1.26-1.55	0.000
Ordinal – probit	6.21		0.000
Ordinal – gompit	6.91		0.000
Nominal – none vs minor	1.44	1.24-1.68	0.000
Nominal – none vs moderate	1.56	1.33-1.83	0.000
Nominal – none vs severe	1.65	1.38-1.97	0.000

Table 15: Logistic regression results for mother unsatisfied with the accommodation for 'other' reasons at age 11

Model	Odds/Z score	95% confidence interval	Significance
Binary logistic	1.32	1.15-1.52	0.000
Ordinal – logistic	1.38	1.23-1.56	0.000
Ordinal – probit	5.22		0.000
Ordinal – gompit	5.79		0.000
Nominal – none vs minor	1.44	1.20-1.72	0.000
Nominal – none vs moderate	1.52	1.26-1.83	0.000
Nominal – none vs severe	1.64	1.33-2.02	0.000

Table 16: Logistic regression results for children living in non-self-contained accommodation at age 11

Model	Odds/Z score	95% confidence interval	Significance
Binary logistic	1.48	1.12-1.95	0.006
Ordinal – logistic	1.37	1.07-1.75	0.013
Ordinal – probit	2.40		0.016
Ordinal – gompit	2.14		0.033
Nominal – none vs minor	0.96	0.65-1.40	0.820
Nominal – none vs moderate	1.40	0.98-2.01	0.065
Nominal – none vs severe	1.53	1.02-2.29	0.039

Table 17: Logistic regression results for child has to share a bed with others at age 11

Model	Odds/Z score	95% confidence interval	Significance
Binary logistic	1.21	1.10-1.32	0.000
Ordinal – logistic	1.32	1.22-1.42	0.000
Ordinal – probit	7.00		0.000
Ordinal – gompit	7.52		0.000
Nominal – none vs minor	1.44	1.28-1.61	0.000
Nominal – none vs moderate	1.31	1.16-1.48	0.000
Nominal – none vs severe	1.61	1.41-1.84	0.000

Table 18: Logistic regression results for mother unsatisfied with accommodation size at age 11

Model	Odds/Z score	95% confidence interval	Significance
Binary logistic	1.24	1.12-1.36	0.000
Ordinal – logistic	1.32	1.21-1.44	0.000
Ordinal – probit	6.36		0.000
Ordinal – gompit	6.96		0.000
Nominal – none vs minor	1.41	1.24-1.59	0.000
Nominal – none vs moderate	1.38	1.21-1.57	0.000
Nominal – none vs severe	1.56	1.35-1.81	0.000

Table 19: Logistic regression results for not having sole access to hot water at age 11

Model	Odds/Z score	95% confidence interval	Significance
Binary logistic	1.28	1.08-1.51	0.004
Ordinal – logistic	1.26	1.08-1.46	0.003
Ordinal – probit	2.99		0.003
Ordinal – gompit	2.38		0.017
Nominal – none vs minor	0.99	0.79-1.24	0.910
Nominal – none vs moderate	1.16	0.92-1.46	0.206
Nominal – none vs severe	1.46	1.14-1.87	0.003

Table 20: Logistic regression results for mother unsatisfied with the garden or outdoor play facilities of the accommodation at age 11

Model	Odds/Z score	95% confidence interval	Significance
Binary logistic	1.27	1.01-1.61	0.044
Ordinal – logistic	1.31	1.06-1.61	0.012
Ordinal – probit	2.59		0.010
Ordinal – gompit	2.36		0.019
Nominal – none vs minor	1.16	0.85-1.58	0.342
Nominal – none vs moderate	1.21	0.88-1.67	0.240
Nominal – none vs severe	1.60	1.14-2.25	0.006

Table 21: Logistic regression results for overcrowding at age 11

Model	Odds/Z score	95% confidence interval	Significance
Binary logistic	1.11	1.04-1.19	0.003
Ordinal – logistic	1.10	1.04-1.17	0.002
Ordinal – probit	3.38		0.001
Ordinal – gompit	1.66		0.097
Nominal – none vs minor	0.93	0.85-1.01	0.096
Nominal – none vs moderate	0.96	0.88-1.06	0.430
Nominal – none vs severe	1.27	1.14-1.41	0.000

Table 22: Logistic regression results for not having sole access to a bath at age 11

Model	Odds/Z score	95% confidence interval	Significance
Binary logistic	1.13	0.99-1.29	0.080
Ordinal – logistic	1.14	1.01-1.29	0.032
Ordinal – probit	2.23		0.026
Ordinal – gompit	1.78		0.075
Nominal – none vs minor	1.04	0.87-1.24	0.702
Nominal – none vs moderate	1.06	0.88-1.28	0.511
Nominal – none vs severe	1.29	1.05-1.58	0.014

Table 23: Logistic regression results for mother unsatisfied with the ownership (eg 'our home') of the accommodation at age 11

Model	Odds/Z score	95% confidence interval	Significance
Binary logistic	1.17	0.87-1.57	0.299
Ordinal – logistic	1.17	0.90-1.51	0.251
Ordinal – probit	1.05		0.290
Ordinal – gompit	1.38		0.167
Nominal – none vs minor	1.22	0.83-1.77	0.310
Nominal – none vs moderate	1.37	0.94-2.02	0.103
Nominal – none vs severe	1.12	0.70-1.80	0.635

Table 24: Logistic regression results for lacking or sharing an indoor toilet at age 11

Model	Odds/Z score	95% confidence interval	Significance
Binary logistic	1.06	0.95-1.18	0.328
Ordinal – logistic	1.06	0.96-1.16	0.273
Ordinal – probit	1.18		0.238
Ordinal – gompit	0.73		0.464
Nominal – none vs minor	0.98	0.85-1.13	0.820
Nominal – none vs moderate	1.00	0.86-1.16	0.980
Nominal – none vs severe	1.13	0.96-1.33	0.148

Table 25: Logistic regression results for not having sole access to a cooker at age 11

Model	Odds/Z score	95% confidence interval	Significance
Binary logistic	0.96	0.61-1.50	0.855
Ordinal – logistic	1.09	0.73-1.60	0.680
Ordinal – probit	0.55		0.585
Ordinal – gompit	0.39		0.695
Nominal – none vs minor	1.19	0.68-2.08	0.543
Nominal – none vs moderate	0.84	0.44-1.60	0.600
Nominal – none vs severe	1.39	0.73-2.64	0.313

Housing deprivation in 1974

Table 26: Logistic regression results for child has to share a bed with others at age 16

Model	Odds/Z score	95% confidence interval	Significance
Binary logistic	1.54	1.34-1.77	0.000
Ordinal – logistic	1.46	1.30-1.65	0.000
Ordinal – probit	6.01		0.000
Ordinal – gompit	5.96		0.000
Nominal – none vs minor	1.17	0.99-1.39	0.066
Nominal – none vs moderate	1.63	1.37-1.94	0.000
Nominal – none vs severe	1.68	1.35-2.08	0.000

Table 27: Logistic regression results for children living in flats at age 16

Model	Odds/Z score	95% confidence interval	Significance
Binary logistic	1.46	1.27-1.67	0.000
Ordinal – logistic	1.45	1.29-1.63	0.000
Ordinal – probit	5.91		0.000
Ordinal – gompit	6.87		0.000
Nominal – none vs minor	1.40	1.19-1.65	0.000
Nominal – none vs moderate	1.81	1.53-2.14	0.000
Nominal – none vs severe	1.43	1.15-1.79	0.002

Table 28: Logistic regression results for overcrowding at age 16

Model	Odds/Z score	95% confidence interval	Significance
Binary logistic	1.32	1.22-1.44	0.000
Ordinal – logistic	1.22	1.14-1.31	0.000
Ordinal – probit	5.61		0.000
Ordinal – gompit	4.64		0.000
Nominal – none vs minor	0.97	0.88-1.07	0.537
Nominal – none vs moderate	1.30	1.17-1.44	0.000
Nominal – none vs severe	1.34	1.18-1.52	0.000

Table 29: Logistic regression results for child living in accommodation with a front door on or above the third floor of the building at age 16

Model	Odds/Z score	95% confidence interval	Significance
Binary logistic	1.31	0.97-1.78	0.077
Ordinal – logistic	1.36	1.05-1.77	0.019
Ordinal – probit	2.23		0.025
Ordinal – gompit	2.61		0.009
Nominal – none vs minor	1.41	0.99-2.01	0.058
Nominal – none vs moderate	1.57	1.07-2.30	0.021
Nominal – none vs severe	1.42	0.86-2.32	0.167

Table 30: Logistic regression results for not having sole access to hot water at age 16

Model	Odds/Z score	95% confidence interval	Significance
Binary logistic	1.48	1.19-1.83	0.000
Ordinal – logistic	1.33	1.10-1.61	0.004
Ordinal –probit	2.86		0.004
Ordinal – gompit	2.20		0.028
Nominal – none vs minor	0.88	0.67-1.17	0.389
Nominal – none vs moderate	1.33	1.00-1.75	0.047
Nominal – none vs severe	1.54	1.11-2.13	0.009

Table 31: Logistic regression results for not having sole access to a bath at age 16

Model	Odds/Z score	95% confidence interval	Significance
Binary logistic	1.39	1.14-1.68	0.000
Ordinal – logistic	1.31	1.11-1.56	0.002
Ordinal – probit	3.18		0.001
Ordinal – gompit	2.48		0.013
Nominal – none vs minor	0.97	0.76-1.24	0.822
Nominal – none vs moderate	1.23	0.95-1.59	0.112
Nominal – none vs severe	1.63	1.22-2.18	0.001

Table 32: Logistic regression results for not having a room to do homework, etc on your own in accommodation at age 16

Model	Odds/Z score	95% confidence interval	Significance
Binary logistic1	0.27	1.13-1.43	0.000
Ordinal – logistic	1.17	1.06-1.30	0.002
Ordinal – probit	3.16		0.002
Ordinal – gompit	2.53		0.011
Nominal – none vs minor	0.96	0.83-1.10	0.519
Nominal – none vs moderate	1.23	1.06-1.42	0.007
Nominal – none vs severe	1.30	1.08-1.56	0.006

Table 33: Logistic regression results for children living in non self-contained accommodation at age 16

Model	Odds/Z score	95% confidence interval	Significance
Binary logistic	1.29	0.83-2.03	0.2536
Ordinal – logistic	1.56	1.07-2.27	0.022
Ordinal – probit	2.34		0.019
Ordinal – gompit	2.66		0.008
Nominal – none vs minor	1.90	1.13-3.19	0.015
Nominal – none vs moderate	1.50	0.82-2.75	0.192
Nominal – none vs severe	2.18	1.12-4.23	0.022

Table 34: Logistic regression results for lacking or sharing an indoor toilet at age 16

Model	Odds/Z score	95% confidence interval	Significance
Binary logistic	1.25	1.05-1.48	0.014
Ordinal – logistic	1.18	1.01-1.37	0.036
Ordinal – probit	2.16		0.031
Ordinal – gompit	1.54		0.123
Nominal – none vs minor	0.94	0.76-1.17	0.575
Nominal – none vs moderate	1.14	0.91-1.43	0.262
Nominal – none vs severe	1.36	1.04-1.77	0.024

Table 35: Logistic regression results for not having sole access to a cooker at age 16

Model	Odds/Z score	95% confidence interval	Significance
Binary logistic	2.09	0.78-5.57	0.141
Ordinal – logistic	1.66	0.69-4.00	0.260
Ordinal – probit	0.94		0.345
Ordinal – gompit	1.66		0.098
Nominal – none vs minor	2.09	0.50-8.73	0.314
Nominal – none vs moderate	4.72	1.25-17.81	0.022
Nominal – none vs severe	-	-	-

Housing deprivation in 1981

Table 36: Logistic regression results for cohort member having been homeless by age 23

Model	Odds/Z score	95% confidence interval	Significance
Binary logistic	1.55	1.31-1.82	0.000
Ordinal – logistic	1.60	1.40-1.83	0.000
Ordinal – probit	6.85		0.000
Ordinal – gompit	6.99		0.000
Nominal – none vs minor	1.48	1.24-1.77	0.000
Nominal – none vs moderate	1.77	1.40-2.22	0.000
Nominal – none vs severe	2.17	1.69-2.79	0.000

Table 37: Logistic regression results for cohort member dissatisfied with present accommodation at age 23

Model	Odds/Z score	95% confidence interval	Significance
Binary logistic	1.24	1.05-1.48	0.012
Ordinal – logistic	1.31	1.15-1.50	0.000
Ordinal – probit	3.96		0.000
Ordinal – gompit	4.10		0.000
Nominal – none vs minor	1.31	1.10-1.55	0.002
Nominal – none vs moderate	1.34	1.06-0.69	0.015
Nominal – none vs severe	1.59	1.22-2.06	0.000

Table 38: Logistic regression results for cohort member living in accommodation with a front door on or above the third floor of the building age 23

Model	Odds/Z score	95% confidence interval	Significance
Binary logistic	0.91	0.70-1.39	0.935
Ordinal – logistic	1.26	0.97-1.64	0.078
Ordinal – probit	1.72		0.085
Ordinal – gompit	2.33		0.020
Nominal – none vs minor	1.61	1.16-2.33	0.005
Nominal – none vs moderate	1.20	0.74-1.95	0.467
Nominal – none vs severe	1.42	0.83-2.42	0.196

Table 39: Logistic regression results for cohort member living in non-self-contained accommodation at age 23

Model	Odds/Z score	95% confidence interval	Significance
Binary logistic	1.39	1.02-1.90	0.036
Ordinal – logistic	1.22	0.95-1.57	0.125
Ordinal – probit	1.44		0.148
Ordinal – gompit	1.27		0.203
Nominal – none vs minor	1.00	0.73-1.38	0.984
Nominal – none vs moderate	1.53	1.03-2.28	0.036
Nominal – none vs severe	1.19	0.71-1.97	0.509

Table 40: Logistic regression results for overcrowding at age 23

Model	Odds/Z score	95% confidence interval	Significance
Binary logistic	1.09	0.86-1.39	0.465
Ordinal – logistic	1.15	0.96-1.38	0.139
Ordinal – probit	1.65		0.099
Ordinal – gompit	1.43		0.151
Nominal – none vs minor	1.14	0.91-1.43	0.259
Nominal – none vs moderate	0.96	0.68-1.35	0.802
Nominal – none vs severe	1.50	1.06-2.11	0.20

Table 41: Logistic regression results for not having sole access to a bath at age 23

Model	Odds/Z score	95% confidence interval	Significance
Binary logistic	1.16	0.93-1.43	0.185
Ordinal – logistic	1.05	0.89-1.24	0.558
Ordinal – probit	0.67		0.505
Ordinal – gompit	0.25		0.806
Nominal – none vs minor	0.93	0.75-1.14	0.485
Nominal – none vs moderate	1.10	0.82-1.46	0.529
Nominal – none vs severe	1.14	0.82-1.59	0.424

Table 42: Logistic regression results for lacking or sharing an indoor toilet at age 23

Model	Odds/Z score	95% confidence interval	Significance
Binary logistic	1.09	0.91-1.32	0.331
Ordinal – logistic	1.03	0.89-1.19	0.681
Ordinal – probit	0.54		0.587
Ordinal – gompit	0.11		0.910
Nominal – none vs minor	0.95	0.79-1.13	0.536
Nominal – none vs moderate	1.01	0.79-1.29	0.930
Nominal – none vs severe	1.15	0.87-1.52	0.324

Table 43: Logistic regression results for not having sole access to a kitchen at age 23

Model	Odds/Z score	95% confidence interval	Significance
Binary logistic	1.07	0.86-1.34	0.550
Ordinal – logistic	1.00	0.84-1.19	0.974
Ordinal – probit	0.01		0.993
Ordinal – gompit	0.10		0.917
Nominal – none vs minor	0.94	0.76-1.16	0.588
Nominal – none vs moderate	1.11	0.83-1.47	0.490
Nominal – none vs severe	0.94	0.66-1.35	0.732

Table 44: Logistic regression results for accommodation below 'bedroom standard' at age 23

Model	Odds/Z score	95% confidence interval	Significance
Binary logistic	1.07	0.94-1.21	0.337
Ordinal – logistic	0.98	0.89-1.09	0.746
Ordinal – probit	0.02		0.982
Ordinal – gompit	0.85		0.397
Nominal – none vs minor	0.89	0.79-1.01	0.065
Nominal – none vs moderate	0.93	0.78-1.10	0.403
Nominal – none vs severe	1.13	0.93-1.37	0.219

Housing deprivation in 1991

Table 45: Logistic regression results for cohort member having been homeless by age 33

Model	Odds/Z score	95% confidence interval	Significance
Binary logistic	1.44	1.18-1.76	0.000
Ordinal – logistic	1.63	1.37-1.95	0.000
Ordinal – probit	5.59		0.000
Ordinal – gompit	6.47		0.000
Nominal – none vs minor	1.93	1.49-2.51	0.000
Nominal – none vs moderate	2.09	1.57-2.79	0.000
Nominal – none vs severe	2.41	1.67-3.48	0.000

Table 46: Logistic regression results for cohort member dissatisfied with the area they live in at age 33

Model	Odds/Z score	95% confidence interval	Significance
Binary logistic	1.49	1.28-1.74	0.000
Ordinal – logistic	1.56	1.37-1.78	0.000
Ordinal – probit	6.74		0.000
Ordinal – gompit	6.53		0.000
Nominal – none vs minor	1.41	1.17-1.69	0.000
Nominal – none vs moderate	1.64	1.33-2.02	0.000
Nominal – none vs severe	2.38	1.83-3.10	0.000

Table 47: Logistic regression results for cohort member dissatisfied with present accommodation at age 33

Model	Odds/Z score	95% confidence interval	Significance
Binary logistic	1.37	1.15-1.64	0.000
Ordinal – logistic	1.50	1.28-1.75	0.000
Ordinal – probit	5.15		0.000
Ordinal – gompit	5.86		0.000
Nominal – none vs minor	1.63	1.31-2.03	0.000
Nominal – none vs moderate	1.81	1.42-2.31	0.000
Nominal – none vs severe	1.93	1.39-2.69	0.000

Table 48: Logistic regression results for accommodation has had serious problems of damp or mould at age 33

Model	Odds/Z score	95% confidence interval	Significance
Binary logistic	1.28	1.14-1.44	0.000
Ordinal – logistic	1.36	1.23-1.51	0.000
Ordinal – probit	6.27		0.000
Ordinal – gompit	5.92		0.000
Nominal – none vs minor	1.31	1.14-1.50	0.000
Nominal – none vs moderate	1.33	1.13-1.56	0.000
Nominal – none vs severe	2.00	1.63-2.45	0.000

Table 49: Logistic regression results for overcrowding at age 33

Model	Odds/Z score	95% confidence interval	Significance
Binary logistic	1.12	0.99-1.27	0.075
Ordinal – logistic	1.23	1.11-1.37	0.000
Ordinal – probit	3.95		0.000
Ordinal – gompit	4.63		0.000
Nominal – none vs minor	1.37	1.19-1.58	0.000
Nominal – none vs moderate	1.31	1.11-1.54	0.001
Nominal – none vs severe	1.44	1.15-1.80	0.002

Table 50: Logistic regression results for cohort member living in accommodation with a front door on or above the third floor of the building at age 33

Model	Odds/Z score	95% confidence interval	Significance
Binary logistic	1.41	0.86-2.30	0.169
Ordinal – logistic	1.47	0.96-2.25	0.079
Ordinal – probit	1.78		0.075
Ordinal – gompit	1.78		0.075
Nominal – none vs minor	1.37	0.75-2.51	0.306
Nominal – none vs moderate	1.57	0.80-3.09	0.187
Nominal – none vs severe	2.03	0.87-4.72	0.100

Table 51: Logistic regression results for cohort member living in non self-contained accommodation at age 33

Model	Odds/Z score	95% confidence interval	Significance
Binary logistic	1.12	0.80-1.57	0.495
Ordinal – logistic	1.15	0.87-1.52	0.332
Ordinal – probit	0.94		0.347
Ordinal – gompit	1.05		0.296
Nominal – none vs minor	1.16	0.80-1.69	0.435
Nominal – none vs moderate	1.23	0.80-1.90	0.348
Nominal – none vs severe	1.20	0.65-2.23	0.559

Table 52: Logistic regression results for not having sole access to a bath at age 33

Model	Odds/Z score	95% confidence interval	Significance
Binary logistic	1.02	0.74-1.41	0.883
Ordinal – logistic	1.13	0.87-1.47	0.359
Ordinal – probit	0.89		0.372
Ordinal – gompit	1.25		0.212
Nominal – none vs minor	1.31	0.92-1.86	0.132
Nominal – none vs moderate	1.21	0.80-1.83	0.378
Nominal – none vs severe	1.17	0.65-2.13	0.596

Table 53: Logistic regression results for not having sole access to a kitchen at age 33

Model	Odds/Z score	95% confidence interval	Significance
Binary logistic	1.01	0.68-1.49	0.967
Ordinal – logistic	1.06	0.77-1.47	0.714
Ordinal – probit	0.25		0.799
Ordinal – gompit	0.60		0.545
Nominal – none vs minor	1.19	0.78-1.83	0.415
Nominal – none vs moderate	1.22	0.74-2.00	0.442
Nominal – none vs severe	0.84	0.37-1.90	0.675

Table 54: Logistic regression results for lacking or sharing an indoor toilet at age 33

Model	Odds/Z score	95% confidence interval	Significance
Binary logistic	0.59	0.17-2.06	0.405
Ordinal – logistic	0.98	0.40-2.41	0.969
Ordinal – probit	0.03		0.973
Ordinal – gompit	0.30		0.764
Nominal – none vs minor	1.87	0.58-6.07	0.298
Nominal – none vs moderate	0.78	0.14-4.28	0.779
Nominal – none vs severe	1.09	0.12-9.78	0.938

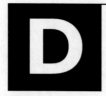

Appendix D: Selected housing and area deprivation indicator questions used in other surveys

About the area you live in

How satisfied are you with this area as a place to live?

1 Very satisfied ☐

2 Fairly satisfied ☐

3 Neither satisfied nor dissatisfied ☐

4 Slightly dissatisfied ☐

5 Very dissatisfied ☐

Source: Survey of English Housing (1996)

Can you tell me how common or uncommon each of these are in this area?

	Very common	Fairly common	Not very common	Not at all common	DK	NA
1 Noisy neighbours or loud parties	☐	☐	☐	☐	☐	☐
2 Graffiti on walls and buildings	☐	☐	☐	☐	☐	☐
3 Teenagers hanging around on the streets	☐	☐	☐	☐	☐	☐
4 Drunks/tramps on the street	☐	☐	☐	☐	☐	☐
5 Rubbish/litter lying around	☐	☐	☐	☐	☐	☐
6 Home and gardens in bad condition	☐	☐	☐	☐	☐	☐
7 Vandalism and deliberate damage to property	☐	☐	☐	☐	☐	☐
8 Insults or attacks to do with someone's race or colour	☐	☐	☐	☐	☐	☐

Source: British Social Attitudes Survey (1996)

And can you tell me how much of a problem are these in your area?

	Very big problem	Fairly big problem	Not very big problem	Not a problem at all	DK	NA
1 Poor street lighting*						
2 Street noise (eg traffic, businesses, factories, etc)†	☐	☐	☐	☐	☐	☐
3 Pollution, grime or other environmental problems caused by traffic or industry†	☐	☐	☐	☐	☐	☐
4 Traffic is a risk to pedestrians and cyclists‡	☐	☐	☐	☐	☐	☐

Source: *British Crime Survey (1994); †European Community Household Panel (1996) (adapted); ‡British Social Attitudes (1993)

From here, how easy would it be for you to get to the following if you needed to?

		a) Easy	b) Not easy
1	Libraries	❐	❐
2	Public sports facilities eg swimming pools	❐	❐
3	Museums and galleries	❐	❐
4	Evening classes	❐	❐
5	Frequent and regular bus services	❐	❐
6	Banks or building societies	❐	❐
7	Chemists	❐	❐
8	Corner shop	❐	❐
9	Medium to large supermarkets	❐	❐
10	Post office	❐	❐
11	Public houses	❐	❐
12	Public hall	❐	❐
13	Petrol stations	❐	❐
14	GP	❐	❐
15	Places of worship	❐	❐
16	Police and other emergency services	❐	❐

Families with children under 5

17	Childcare facilities such as nurseries or playgroups	❐	❐
18	Play facilities for children to play safely nearby	❐	❐

Families with school-age children

19	Schools	❐	❐
20	Youth clubs/after school clubs	❐	❐

Source: adapted from the *Breadline Britain* in the 1990s survey, Housing Attitudes Survey (1992), Rural Development Commission (1992), the HEFCW Survey of Rural Services (1995-96)

How satisfied are you with this accommodation?

1 Very satisfied ❐
2 Fairly satisfied ❐
3 Neither satisfied nor dissatisfied ❐
4 Slightly dissatisfied ❐
5 Very dissatisfied ❐

Source: Survey of English Housing (1996)

Would you describe the state of repair of your home as good, adequate or poor?

1 Good ❐
2 Adequate ❐
3 Poor ❐
9 Don't know ❐

Source: *Breadline Britain* in the 1990s survey

Do you have any of the following problems with your accommodation?

Yes	❐
No	❐
Don't Know	❐

Source: Breadline Britain in the 1990s survey

		Yes	No	Don't know
1	Shortage of space	❐	❐	❐
2	Too dark, not enough light	❐	❐	❐
3	Lack of adequate heating facilities	❐	❐	❐
4	Leaky roof	❐	❐	❐
5	Damp walls, floors, foundations, etc	❐	❐	❐
6	Rot in window frames or floors	❐	❐	❐
7	Mould	❐	❐	❐
8	No place to sit outside, eg a terrace or garden	❐	❐	❐
9	Other	❐	❐	❐

Source: European Community Household Panel Survey (1996), HEA: Health and Lifestyles – Black and Minority Ethnic Groups (1994)

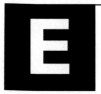

Appendix E: Analysis of response bias in the NCDS

In order for longitudinal research to be accurate, the continued representativeness of the original sample is clearly important. The overall response to the NCDS follow-ups has remained satisfactorily high as a per cent of those known to be alive and living in this country, although it has declined from 98% in 1958 to 70% in 1991. The lower response at the NCDS sweep 4 and NCDS sweep 5 was largely due to difficulties in tracing the cohort members, although refusals had increased from 0.4% at NCDS sweep 1 to 11% at NCDS sweep 5. The reduction in the response rate introduces the possibility of bias in the remaining sample. Thus one has to question whether the cohort members interviewed in NCDS5 at the age of 33 were representative of the original cohort and, thereby, more generally of people of about that age in Britain. Fogelman (1976) found that up to the age of 16, differences between cohort members in NCDS sweep 1 and NCDS sweep 3 were generally small or non-existent in relation to indices such as social class, region and measures of physical development. There was, however, evidence of a slight under-representation of those who might broadly be termed 'disadvantaged' in relation to family, housing and financial circumstances. These included children receiving special education at the age of 11, children who were illegitimate and children who had been in voluntary society or local authority care by the age of 7. Further small differences were found in test scores, with those children without data at age 16 having lower reading, mathematics and general ability scores at age 11. A more serious bias was found in relation to immigrant status and ethnicity: 16-year-olds of Caribbean origin were under-represented by about one third, those from the Indian subcontinent by about one quarter and those from Ireland by about one tenth.

Table 1 details the response bias in NCDS sweep 5 compared with earlier follow-ups. It reveals a similar picture to that which Fogelman found for the cohort aged 16. The greatest losses in NCDS sweep 5 were for ethnic minority and immigrant groups, particularly those of Afro-Caribbean appearance and those from the West Indies. Also under-represented in the NCDS sweep 5 were male respondents, 'low achievement' groups and those with 'low aspirations', those who were 'handicapped', who had been in voluntary society or local authority care in childhood, who came from the lower social classes or who were brought up in poorer housing conditions.

A second method of analysing response bias is to compare distributions on key variables with those variables available from other sources. Table 2 details some of the key characteristics of the NCDS sweep 5 population in comparison with those of other national surveys. In general the results are encouraging: the differences are "generally quite small given the differences in age and age banding, survey timing and definition" (Shepherd, 1995, p 187).

Table 1: Response bias in NCDS sweep 5 compared with earlier follow-ups

Variable	% bias
Mother born in the West Indies	-50.00
Father born in the West Indies	-45.45
Child's ethnic group is Afro-Caribbean	-45.45
Parents don't want the child to stay on at school	-17.02
Low maths score at age 11	-16.10
Low reading score at age 11	-15.50
Any child receives free school meals (1974)	-15.69
Family in financial hardship (1974)	-12.50
Child ever in care 1958-65	-12.50
Tenure 'private rented' (1969)	-9.09
Family share one or more housing amenities (1969)	-8.00
Child reported 'handicapped' at age 16	-6.58
Male respondents	-3.91
Father's social class in 1974 – manual	-3.33

Source: Shepherd (1995, p 185)

Table 2: Some key characteristics of the NCDS sweep 5 population in comparison with those of the General Household Survey (GHS) and the New Earnings Survey (NES)

Marital status	GHS 1989 (age 30-34)	GHS 1991 (age 25-34)	GHS 1991 (age 35-44)	NCDS sweep 5 (age 33)
Single	13	23	8	12
Married	72	60	77	71
Cohabiting	9	11	5	10
Separated	2	2	2	2
Divorced	4	4	6	5
Widowed	<1	0	1	<1

Economic activity	GHS 1991 (age 25-34)	NCDS sweep 5 (age 33)
Men		
Working	87	90
Unemployed	10	6
Inactive	3	4
Women		
Working	64	68
Unemployed	5	2
Inactive	31	30

Gross weekly pay (£)	GHS 1989 (age 30-39)	NES 1991 (age 30-39)	NCDS sweep 5 (age 33)
Men			
Median	253	-	285
Mean	-	341	320
Women			
Median	179	-	231
Mean	-	252	257

Tenure	GHS 1991 (age 30-44)	NCDS sweep 5 (age 33)
Own/buying	75	75
Renting from local authority, new town, housing association	19	20
Renting privately	4	4
Other	2	1

Ethnic group	GHS 1989 (age 25-44)	NCDS sweep 5 (age 33)
White	94	98
Indian	1	1
Pakistani/Bangladeshi	1	<1
Black/Caribbean	1	1
Other	2	<1

Source: Shepherd (1995, p 188)